THE SIRTFOOD DIET:

D1277717

BEGINNER'S GUIDE FOR FAST WEIGHT LOSS, BURN FAT AND ACTIVATES THE METABOLISM WITH THE HELP OF SIRT FOODS. INCLUDES DELICIOUS AND HEALTHY RECIPES FOR YOUR MEAL PLAN.

Lisa Middleton

Table of Contents

Introduction

The sirtfood diet depends on the possibility that specific nourishments actuate sirtuins in your body, which are particular proteins guessed to receive different rewards, from shielding cells in your body from aggravation to switching maturing. Nourishments permitted on the eating regimen incorporate green tea, dim chocolate, apples, organic citrus products, parsley, turmeric, kale, blueberries, tricks and red wine.

On the authority Sirt food diet site, defenders clarify that the eating regimen has two "simple" stages. Stage one is seven days with every day comprising of three sort food green juices and one dinner loaded up with sirtfoods — a sum of 1,000 calories. You may be somewhat less starving on days four through seven when you're permitted to expand your admission to 1,500 calories with two green juices and two dinners.

Stage two isn't significantly more encouraging. This stage goes on for about fourteen days, in which you are allowed to have three "adjusted" sirtfood-rich suppers every day notwithstanding your one extraordinary green juice. The objective during this time is to advance further weight reduction. While the advantages of sirtuins appear to be encouraging, the sirtfood diet is promoted up 'til now another approach to "shed seven pounds in seven days!" And you know at this point outrageous weight control plans simply don't work that way.

What seems like a tidbit lifted directly from a science fiction motion picture, a 'sirtfood' is nourishment high in sirtuin activators? Sirtuins are a sort of protein which shield the cells in our bodies from biting the dust or getting aggravated through sickness, however, investigate has likewise demonstrated they can help manage your digestion, increment muscle and consume fat.

Two big-name nutritionists working for a private exercise centre in the UK built up the Sirtfood Diet. They promote the eating routine as a regular new eating routine and wellbeing plan that works by turning on your "thin quality." This eating regimen depends on to inquire about on sirtuins (SIRTs), a gathering of seven proteins found in the body that has been appeared to control an assortment of capacities, including digestion, irritation and life expectancy. Specific individual plant mixes might have the option to expand the degree of these proteins in the body, and nourishments containing them have been named "sirtfoods."

The Sirtfood Diet book was first distributed in the U.K. in 2016. Be that as it may, the U.S. arrival of the book, coming this March, has started the greater interest in the arrangement. The eating routine started getting publicity when Adele debuted her slimmer figure at the Billboard Music Awards last May. Her coach, Pete Geracimo, is a huge aficionado of the eating routine and says the vocalist shed 30 pounds from following a Sirt food diet.

Sirtfoods are wealthy in supplements that actuate a supposed "thin quality" called sirtuin. As indicated by Goggins and Matten, the "thin quality" is initiated when a lack of vitality is made after you confine calories. Sirtuins got fascinating to the nourishment world in 2003 when specialists found that resveratrol, a compound found in red wine, had a similar impact on life range as calorie limitation however it was accomplished without diminishing admission.

In the 2015 pilot study (led by Goggins and Matten) testing the viability of sirtuins, the 39 members lost a normal of seven pounds in seven days. Those outcomes sound noteworthy, yet it's critical to understand this is a small example size concentrated over a brief timeframe. Weight reduction specialists additionally have their questions about the elevated guarantees. "The cases made are extremely theoretical and extrapolate from examines which were generally centred around basic life forms (like yeast) at the cell level. What occurs at the cell level doesn't mean what occurs in the human body at the large scale level," says Adrienne Youdim, M.D., the executive of the Center for Weight Loss and Nutrition in Beverly Hills, CA.

What nourishments are high in sirtuins?

The book contains a rundown of the leading 20 nourishments that are high in sirtuins, which sounds more like a drifting nourishment list than another, advanced eating routine. Models include arugula, chilies, espresso, green tea, Medjool dates, red wine, turmeric, pecans, and the wellbeing cognizant top pick kale. Dr Youdim takes note of that while the nourishments being advanced are stable, they won't advance weight reduction all alone.

The fundamental reason of the Sirtfood Diet is that sure nourishments, named "sirtfoods," can emulate the demonstrated advantages of caloric limitation and fasting by method for actuating sirtuins—proteins in the body (going from SIRT1 to SIRT7) that manage natural pathways, turn certain qualities on and off, and help shield cells from age-related decay. Enactment of SIRT1, for instance, has been appeared in some lab and creature concentrates on initiating the development of new mitochondria, expanding life length, and improve oxidative digestion, which may bolster weight reduction and support.

Since fasting and extreme caloric limitation is extremely hard (and frequently, not fitting), Goggins and Matten built up their dietary arrangement—concentrated on eating heaps of "sirtfoods"— as a more straightforward method to invigorate the body's sirtuin qualities (in some cases alluded to as "thin qualities") and in this way increase weight reduction and advance by and broad wellbeing.

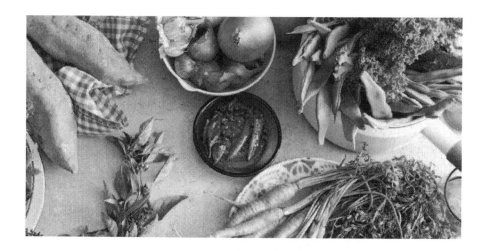

What makes something a "sirtfood"?

Green tea, berries, cocoa powder, turmeric, kale, onions, parsley, arugula, chilies, espresso, red wine, pecans, escapades, buckwheat, and olive oil. These nourishments contain explicit polyphenol mixes (quercetin, resveratrol, kaempferol, and so on.) that have, truth be told, been found in logical investigations to increment sirtuin action. Along these lines, right now, diet is at any rate to some degree dependent on science.

The issue, notwithstanding, is that these nourishments may not contain adequate degrees of these polyphenols to enact sirtuins in any meaningful manner. A large number of the examinations connecting polyphenol mixes to expanded sirtuin action have just been done on exceptionally focused types of these mixes.

Chapter 1   The Science Behind It All

The sirtfood diet can't be classified as low-carb or low-fat. This diet is quite different from its many precursors while advocating many of the same things: the ingestion of fresh, plant-based foods. As the name implies, this is a sirtuin based diet, but what are sirtuins and why have you never heard about them before?

There are seven sirtuin proteins – SIRT-1 to SIRT-7[1]. They can be found throughout your cells and the cells of every animal on the planet. Sirtuins are found in almost every living organism and in almost every part of the cell, controlling what goes on. Supplement company Elysium Health, likens the body's cells to an office with sirtuins acting as the CEO, helping the cells react to internal and external changes. They govern what is done, when it's done, and who does is.

Of the seven sirtuins, one works in your cell's cytoplasm, three in the cell's mitochondria, and another three in the cell's nucleus. They have a wide number of jobs to perform, but mostly they remove acetyl groups from other proteins. These acetyl groups signal that the protein they are attached to is available to perform its function. Sirtuins remove the available flag and get the protein ready to use.

Sirtuins sound pretty crucial to your body's normal function, so why is that you've never heard of them before?

The first sirtuin to be discovered was SIR2, a gene discovered in the 1970s which controlled the ability of fruit flies to mate. It wasn't until the 1990s that scientists discovered other, similar proteins, in almost every form of life. Every organism had a different number of sirtuins – bacteria has one and yeast has five. Experiments on mice show they have the same number as humans, seven.

Sirtuins have been shown to prolong life in yeast and in mice. There is, so far, no evidence of the same effect in human beings, however, these sirtuins are present in almost every form of life and many scientists are hopeful that if organisms as far apart as yeast and mice can see the same effect from sirtuin activation, this may also extend to humans.

In addition to sirtuins, our bodies need another substance called noicotineamide adenine dinucleotide for cells to function properly. Elysium (see above) likens this substance to the money a company needs to keep operating. Like any CEO, a sirtuin can only keep the company working properly if the cash flow is sufficient. NAD+ was first discovered in 1906. You get your supply of NAD+ from your diet by eating foods made up the building blocks of NAD+.

Fun Facts about Sirtuins:

1. Mice that have been engineered to have high levels of SIRT-1 are both more active and leaner than normal, while mice that lack SIRT-1 altogether are fatter and more prone to various metabolic conditions.

2. Add the fact that levels of SIRT-1 are much lower in obese people than in those of a "healthy" weight and the case for the importance of sirtuins in weight loss becomes compelling.

3. By making a permanent change to your diet and adding the best sirtfoods to your eating plan, the authors of the sirtfood diet believe everyone can achieve better health, all without losing muscle mass.

To Sum Up

Exercise and calorie restriction are both sources of stress which encourage our bodies to adapt to changing circumstances. If the stress becomes too great the result can be injury, the body can even die, but at lower levels, we adapt and this temporary, low-level stress is key to many physiological changes.

For example, stress on muscles, enough but not too much, is what makes the body increase muscle mass.

Similarly, the authors of the sirtfood diet found that it is when the body is stressed, by exercise or low-calorie intake, that the effect of sirtuins kicks in and it is this effect that can be reproduced by a diet rich in SIRT foods.

Is this the diet for you?

Any diet plan you adopt involves some level of expense and inconvenience. It may also involve risk. Anyone can write a diet book, as there is no need to have the diet medically approved. That's one reason why all diets start by suggesting you consult a doctor. One thing you can do is look at the qualifications of the diet's author.

The authors of the sirtfood diet are not TV personalities or reality stars. They have genuine scientific knowledge of the subject and both have Master's degrees to prove it.

Aidan Goggins is a pharmacist, with a degree in pharmacy and a Master's degree in Nutritional Medicine. Glen Matten trained at the Institute for Optimum Nutrition before completing his Master's degree in nutritional medicine.

The sirtfood diet is not their first collaboration. In 2012, they wrote *"The Health Delusion,"* a book that attacked many of the "long held truths" of the diet and health industry. As a result, they received the consumer health book of the year award by the Medical Journalists Association.

Having reviewed the literature and asked the big question: "What would happen if we ate sirtfoods? Would there be weight loss?" they went on to ask: "What would happen to muscle mass, which is usually lost during almost any diet?"

To find the answers, the authors conducted a trial in an exclusive health spa near London in the UK. There were 40 participants. 39 completed the trial. Because the trial was carried out at a health spa, the authors had complete control over the food eaten by the participants. Note that this is not always the case in "medical" trials where the participants report what they ate.

The discovery and history of sirtuins

There were different quantities of sirtuins in every creature. For instance, yeast has five sirtuins, microscopic organisms have one, mice have seven, and people have seven.

The way that sirtuins were found across species implies they were "saved" with development. Qualities that are "rationed" have all-inclusive capacities in numerous or all species. What was at this point to be known, however, was the means by which significant sirtuins would end up being.

In 1991, Elysium fellow benefactor and MIT scholar Leonard Guarente, nearby alumni understudies Nick Austriaco and Brian Kennedy, led trials to all the more likely see how yeast matured. By some coincidence, Austriaco attempted to develop societies of different yeast strains from tests he had put away in his ice chest for quite a long time, which made a distressing domain for the strains. Just a portion of these strains could develop from here, yet Guarente and his group identified an example: The strains of yeast that endure the best in the cooler were likewise the longest lived. This gave direction to Guarente so he could concentrate exclusively on these long-living strains of yeast.

This prompted the identification of SIR2 as a quality that advanced life span in yeast. It's critical to note more research is required on SIR2's belongings in people. The Guarente lab consequently found that expelling SIR2 abbreviated yeast life range significantly, while in particular, expanding the quantity of duplicates of the SIR2 quality from one to two expanded the life length in yeast. In any case, what initiated SIR2 normally presently couldn't seem to be found.

This is the place acetyl bunches become possibly the most important factor. It was at first idea that SIR2 may be a deacetylating protein — which means it expelled those acetyl gatherings — from different atoms, yet nobody knew if this were valid since all endeavors to show this movement in a test tube demonstrated negative. Guarente and his group had the option to find that SIR2 in yeast could just deacetylate different proteins within the sight of the coenzyme NAD+, nicotinamide adenine dinucleotide.

In Guarente's own words: "Without NAD+, SIR2 sits idle. That was the basic finding on the circular segment of sirtuin science."

Chapter 2   Sirtuins, Fasting, And Metabolic Activities

SIRT1, just like other SIRTUINS family, is protein NAD+ dependent deacetylases that are associated with cellular metabolism. All sirtuins, including SIRT1 important for sensing energy status and in protection against metabolic stress. They coordinate cellular response towards Caloric Restriction (CR) in an organism. SIRT1 diverse location and allows cells to easily sense changes in the level of energy anywhere in the mitochondria, nucleus, and cytoplasm. Associated with metabolic health through deacetylation of several target proteins such as muscles, liver, endothelium, heart, and adipose tissue.

SIRT1, SIRT6, and SIRT7 are localized in the nucleus where they take part in the deacetylation of customers to influence gene expression epigenetically. SIRT2 is located in the cytosol, while SIRT3, SIRT4, and SIRT5 are located in the mitochondria where they regulate metabolic enzyme activities as well as moderate oxidative stress.

SIRT1, as most studies with regards to metabolism, aid in mediating the physiological adaptation to diets. Several studies have shown the impact of sirtuins on Caloric Restriction. Sirtuins deacetylase non-histone proteins that define pathways involved during the metabolic adaptation when there are metabolic restrictions. Caloric Restriction, on the other hand, causes the induction of expression of SIRT1 in humans. Mutations that lead to loss of function in some sirtuins genes can lead to a reduction in the outputs of caloric restrictions. Therefore, sirtuins have the following metabolic functions:

Regulation in the liver

The Liver regulates the body glucose homeostasis. During fasting or caloric restriction, glucose level becomes low, resulting in a sudden shift in hepatic metabolism to glycogen breakdown and then to gluconeogenesis to maintain glucose supply as well as ketone body production to mediate the deficit in energy. Also, during caloric restriction or fasting, there is muscle activation and liver oxidation of fatty acids produced during lipolysis in white adipose tissue. For this switch to occur, there are several transcription factors involved to adapt to energy deprivation. SIRT1 intervenes during the metabolic switch to see the energy deficit.

At the initial stage of the fasting that is the post glycogen breakdown phase, there is the production of glucagon by the pancreatic alpha cells to active gluconeogenesis in the Liver through the cyclic amp response element-binding protein (CREB), and CREB regulated transcription coactivator 2 (CRTC2), the coactivator. Is the fasting gets prolonged, the effect is cancelled out and is being replaced by SIRT1 mediated CRTC2 deacetylase resulting in targeting of the coactivator for ubiquitin/proteasome-mediated destruction? SIRT1, on the other hand, initiates the next stage of gluconeogenesis through acetylation and activation of peroxisome proliferator-activated receptor coactivator one alpha, which is the coactivator necessary for fork head box O1. In addition to the ability of SIRT1 to support gluconeogenesis, coactivator one alpha is required during the mitochondrial biogenesis necessary for the liver to accommodate the reduction in energy status. SIRT1 also activates fatty acid oxidation through deacetylation and activation of the nuclear receptor to increase energy production. SIRT1, when involved in acetylation and repression of glycolytic enzymes such as phosphoglycerate mutate 1, can lead to shutting down of the production of energy through glycolysis. SIRT6, on the other hand, can be served as a co-repressor for hypoxia-inducible Factor 1 Alpha to repress glycolysis. Since SIRT6 can transcriptionally be induced by SIRT1, sirtuins can coordinate the duration of time for each fasting phase.

Aside from glucose homeostasis, the liver also overtakes in lipid and cholesterol homeostasis during fasting. When there are caloric restrictions, the synthesis of fat and cholesterol in the liver is turned off, while lipolysis in the white adipose tissue commences. The SIRT1, upon fasting, causes acetylation of steroid regulatory element-binding protein (SREBP) and targets the protein to destroy the ubiquitin-professor system. The result is that fat cholesterol synthesis will repress. During the regulation of cholesterol homeostasis, SIRT1 regulates oxysterol receptor, thereby, assisting the reversal of cholesterol transport from peripheral tissue through upregulation of the oxysterol receptor target gene ATP-binding cassette transporter A1 (ABCA1).

Further modulation of the cholesterol regulatory loop can be achieved via bile acid receptor, that's necessary for the biosynthesis of cholesterol catabolic and bile acid pathways. SIRT6 also participates in the regulation of cholesterol levels by repressing the expression and post-translational cleavage of SREBP1/2, into the active form. Furthermore, in the circadian regulation of metabolism, SIRT1 participates through the regulation of cell circadian clock.

Mitochondrial SIRT3 is crucial in the oxidation of fatty acid in mitochondria. Fasting or caloric restrictions can result in up-regulation of activities and levels of SIRT3 to aid fatty acid oxidation through deacetylation of long-chain specific acyl-CoA dehydrogenase. SIRT3 can also cause activation of ketogenesis and the urea cycle in the liver.

SIRT1 also Add it in the metabolic regulation in the muscle and white adipose tissue. Fasting causes an increase in the level of SIRT1, leading to deacetylation of coactivator one alpha, which in turn causes genes responsible for fat oxidation to get activated. The reduction in energy level also activates AMPK, which will activate the expression of coactivator one alpha. The combined effects of the two processes will give rise to increased mitochondrial biogenesis together with fatty acid oxidation in the muscle.

Chapter 3   Ways to Follow the Sirtfood Diet Plans

Eating some quality foods will improve your "skinny gene" pathways and enables you to shed some unnecessary weight in seven days. Food such as kale, dark chocolate, and wine has a natural compounds known as polyphenols that look likes the results of fitness workout and fasting. Strawberries, cinnamon, as well as turmeric are also strong **sirtfoods**. These foods will activate the sirtuin steps or potential to help improve weight loss.

There are 2 phases to follow the sirtfood diet:

PHASE 1 OF THE SIRTFOOD DIET

All through the first 3 days, calorie consumption is reduced to 1,000 calories (that is more than on a 5:2 fasting day). The diet involves 3 Sirtfood-full of green juices and 1 Sirtfood filled meal and 2 serves of dark chocolate.

For the remaining 4 days calories intake has to be increased to 1, 500 calories and daily day the diet should involves 2 Sirtfood- filled green juices and 2 Sirtfood-rich meals.

In the early first stage "The phase 1 stage" you are not permitted to drink any alcohol, but you are free to take water and green tea.

PHASE 2 OF THE SIRTFOOD DIET

Phase 2 does not center on calorie intake reduction. Daily intake involves 3 Sirtfood-rich foods and 1 green juice, and the alternative of 1 or 2 Sirtfood crunch snacks, if necessary.

In the second phase 2 you are permitted to take red wine, but not too much (they advise you to take 2-3 glasses of red wine weekly), and also water, tea, coffee and green tea.

After the Diet

You may replicate these two phases as much you desired for additional weight loss.

However, you are advised to continue "sirtifying" your diet at the end of completing these phases by including sirtfoods frequently into your meals.

There are a variations of Sirtfood Diet manuals that has several recipes rich in sirtfoods. You can also add sirtfoods in your foods as a snack or in recipes you have previously use. In addition, you are advised to continue taking the green juice daily.

In this manner, the Sirtfood Diet will be more of a way of lifestyle adjustment than a one-time diet.

Diet to activate sirtuins and promote health

It's apparently no accident that some of the individuals with long lifespan and healthiest populations in the world eat diets that are rich in these sirtuin activating foods, examples are those in the Mediterranean and parts of Asia. The Mediterranean diet includes polyphenol rich fruits, veggies, olive oil including red wine. The Asian diet is rich in isoflavones present in soya beans and epigallactins from green tea.

Acquiring several of these health developing foods into your diet is proportionately easy. They can be included into many diets and even compound to make super-sirt meals!

Below are some grate ideas you can get started with

- Make use olive oil for frying or roasting veggies or vegetables and salad dressings.

- Ensure to own a jar of olives handy to snack on and include olives to salads or cooked meals. Tapenade usually makes a great topping for rye breads.

- Exchange usual tea and coffee for green tea. Include a press of lemon for extra interest.

- Miso alternatively can be used rather than stock cubes to flavor soups and stews. Milder light colored miso may be used as a spread. Miso soup makes a great snack or soft meal if presented with salad or bread.

- Include tofu or tempeh to stir fries. Mix silken tofu into soups, immerse and creamy desserts.

- Put berries, blackcurrants to muesli, smoothies and juices. Fresh yoghurt as well as fresh berries ensure a healthy snack or dessert.

- Take your greens. Cabbage and broccoli are outstanding support to any meal and can also be included to stir fries, curries, stews and casseroles.

- Enrich up your life with turmeric and other spices. Don't restrict your input of seasonings to curries, include them to grains and vegetables.

- Include cacao powder to smoothies and desserts too. Dredge cacao nibs on salads or include to trail mixes.

- Apples are the ideal handy snack. Make sure you have one with you most times.

- Buckwheat macaroni can be made as a tasty gluten complimentary option to wheat pasta and buckwheat flour can be made also in baked products or to stiffer sauces. Buckwheat is also a great alternative that goes well with salads combined with roasted vegetables and toasted nuts.

Top 20 sirtfoods

In alphabetical order

1.   Arugula (Rocket)

2.   Buckwheat

3.   Capers

4.   Celery

5.   Chilies

6.   Cocoa

7.   Coffee

8.   Extra Virgin Olive Oil

9.   Garlic

10.   Green Tea (especially Matcha)

11.   Kale

12.   Medjool Dates

13.   Parsley

14.   Red Endive

15.   Red Onions

16.   Red Wine

17. Soy

18. Strawberries

19. Turmeric

20. Walnuts

Chapter 4   Sirtfood Green Juice

Recipe & cooking advice

When trying to cook with the sirtfoods most of the ingredients you should be familiar with already. However there are a few which will be new.

Matcha is green tea, but in a powdered form. You're unlikely to be able to buy it from the shelves of your local supermarket, but it will be available from health specialist stores or from online retailers. Matcha is generally produced in China and Japan, where it is a traditional beverage, so you should expect to order from overseas.

It is better if you can buy Matcha from Japan, as Matcha from China may have forms of pollution and impurities due to the environment. Matcha green tea is used in Zen ceremonies in Japan and it is even better for you than regular green tea. The unique nature of Matcha green tea originates from how it is grown. Matcha is grown almost entirely in dark shadowy environments, whilst green tea is usually grown in bright sunshine.

Matcha is also ground into a power using a mill, rather than being cut into small leaves and added as an infusion.

Lovage is another ingredient you probably have never heard of. Lovage is an herb, but one that hasn't been used by our culinary society for over 100 years. It can be bought, but it is more practical to grow your own. Lovage plants are low maintenance – you should be able to plant the seeds in a regular pot, put it on the windowsill in your house, water it once a day and see growth in a few weeks. Lovage seeds will be available from most garden centers (or you can buy an already thriving plant).

Additionally, you may or may not have heard of buckwheat. Buckwheat is a grain that is high in protein, carbohydrate and sirtuin. However, other foods made from buckwheat, such as buckwheat pasta or soba noodles will need to either be bought online or sourced from a specialist store.

Small variations to the main meal recipes provided later can help make them more palatable. For example, Bird's-eye or Thai Chilies are more potent than the chilies typically used in the Western diet. Owing to this if you are not well-acquainted with spicy foods; you should reduce the amount you add into your recipes to begin with. Try half the recommended value, ensuring you de-seed the chili as the seeds themselves are rather spicy.

Miso is a type of soya-bean paste, which is used for flavoring in eastern dishes. Miso comes in multiple flavors, with the lighter colored variants being sweeter than the darker colors. You can experiment with what flavor suits you best. On a similar vein, the potency of the miso varies between the different colors (white, yellow, red & brown), so you might want to lower or increase the amount of miso you use to get the taste just right.

Buckwheat should be washed before it is cooked, by placing it in a sieve and rinsing it with water. Flat leaf parsley is preferable to curly leaf, but the latter is acceptable if you cannot source the former.

Finally, feel free to season and add salt and pepper as necessary, although the recipes are intended to be tasty without additional flavoring.

Green Juice

Alright, let's finally get down to business. The first three days of the hyper-success phase allows you to consume up to 1000 calories from 3* sirtfood green juices and 1*main meal. The juices are especially prominent in the diet because they allow you to consume more sirtfoods for a lower calorie cost.

So what is this fabled 'green juice?? ?' The green juice is simply a blend of some of the sirtuin superfoods, with a few added healthy ingredients for taste and to promote digestion and absorption. The green juice is made with Kale, Rocket, Parsley, Lovage, Green Celery (including leaves) and Match green tea.

The exact recipe is as follows;

Ingredients:

75g Kale

30g Rocket

5g Flat-leaf parsley

5g Lovage leaves

150g Celery

½ a green apple

Juice of ½ a lemon

½ level tsp Matcha

Whilst these are the official measurements, you can generally approximate the recipe as follows;

2 handfuls of kale

1 handful of rocket

A pinch of parsley

A pinch of lovage

3 large celery stalks

½ a green apple

Juice of ½ a lemon

½ level tsp Matcha

Directions:

Using the handful measurement also helps you to adjust how you make the green juice – people with larger bodies (and larger hands) will receive slightly more of each ingredient, which should ensure that they are getting proportionally enough.

Start making the green juice by juicing the leafy greens and herbs – you should be aiming to produce about 50ml of liquid. Juicers vary in their ability to process the greens, so you might need multiple processing attempts to generate the juice.

Next add the celery and apple, juicing once more. Squeeze in the lemon juice and blend again. You should have approximately 1 cup (250ml) of juice to work with.

Separate the juice into two equal sized portions. Toss in the Matcha to one portion, stirring vigorously. Matcha is only added to the morning and the midday juice as it contains noticeable amounts of caffeine and may keep you awake in the evening. After the Matcha has been absorbed, pour the two portions back together and stir.

Your juice is now ready. You may want to add some water, according to your own sense of taste. There is no need to make the juice from scratch every time you want it – you can produce batches, which should stay fresh and not lose any of their value for up to 3 days, as long as you keep them chilled.

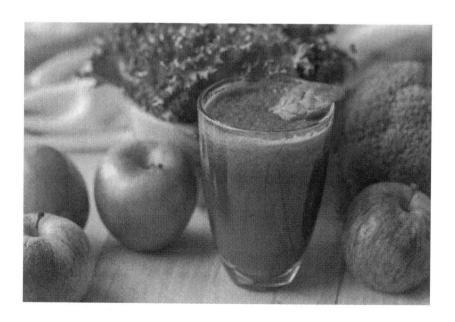

Chapter 5   Phase 1 and Phase 2

Phase 1: 7 pounds in seven days

Monday: 3 green juices

- Breakfast: water + tea or espresso + a cup of green juice;

- Lunch: green juice

- Snack: a square of dark chocolate;

- Dinner: Sirt meal

- After dinner: a square of dark chocolate.

Drink the juices at three distinct times of the day (for example, in the morning as soon as you wake up, mid-morning and mid-afternoon) and choose the normal or vegan dish: pan-fried oriental prawns with buckwheat spaghetti or miso and tofu with sesame glaze and sautéed vegetables (vegan dish)

Tuesday: 3 green juices

- Breakfast: water + tea or espresso + a cup of green juice

- Lunch: 2 green juices before dinner;

- Snack: a square of dark chocolate;

- Dinner: Sirt meal

- After dinner: a square of dark chocolate.

Welcome to day 2 of the Sirtfood Diet. The formula is identical to that of the first day, and the only thing that changes is the solid meal. Today you will also have dark chocolate, and the same goes for tomorrow. This food is so wonderful that we don't need an excuse to eat it.

To earn the title of a "Sirt food", chocolate must be at least 85 percent cocoa. And even among the various types of chocolate with this percentage, not all of them are the same. Often this product is treated with an alkalizing agent (this is the so-called "Dutch process") to reduce its acidity and give it a darker color. Unfortunately, this process greatly reduces the flavonoids activating sirtuins, compromising their health benefits. Lindt Excellence 85% chocolate, is not subjected to the Dutch process and is therefore often recommended.

On day 2, capers are also included in the menu. Despite what many may think, they are not fruits, but buds that grow in Mediterranean countries and are picked by hand. They are fantastic Sirt foods because they are very rich in the nutrients kaempferol and quercetin. From the point of view of flavour, they are tiny concentrates of taste. If you've never used them, don't feel intimidated. You will see, they will taste amazingly if combined with the right ingredients, and they will give an unmistakable and inimitable aroma to your dishes.

On the second day, you will intake: 3 green Sirt juices and one solid meal (normal or vegan).

Drink the juices at three distinct times of the day (for example, when you wake up in the morning, mid-morning and mid-afternoon) and choose either the normal or the vegan dish: Turkey escalope with capers, parsley, and sage on spiced cauliflower couscous or curly kale and red onion Dahl with buckwheat (vegan dish)

Wednesday: 3 green juices

- Breakfast: water + tea or espresso + a cup of green juice

- Lunch: 2 green juices before dinner;

- Snack: a square of dark chocolate;

- Dinner: Sirt meal

- After dinner: a square of dark chocolate.

You are now on the third day, and even if the format is once again identical to that of days 1 and 2, so the time has come to flavor everything with a fundamental ingredient. For thousands of years, chili has been a fundamental element of the gastronomic experiences of the whole world.

As for the effects on health, we have already seen that its spiciness is perfect for activating sirtuins and stimulating the metabolism. The applications of chili are endless, and therefore represent an easy way to consume a Sirt food regularly.

If you are not a big expert of chili, we recommend the Bird's Eye (sometimes called Thai chili), because it is the best for sirtuins.

This is the last day you will consume three green juices a day; tomorrow, you will switch to two. We, therefore, take this opportunity to browse other drinks that you can have during the diet. We all know that green tea is good for health, and water is naturally very good, but what about coffee? More than half of people drink at least one coffee a day, but always with a trace of guilt because some say that it is a vice and an unhealthy habit. This is absolutely untrue; studies show that coffee is a real treasure trove of beneficial plant substances. That's why coffee drinkers run the least risk of getting diabetes, certain forms of cancer, and neurodegenerative diseases. Furthermore, not only is coffee, not a toxin, it protects the liver and makes it even healthier!

On the third day, you will intake 3 green Sirt juices and 1 one solid meal (normal or vegan, see below).

Drink the juices at three distinct times of the day (for example, in the morning as soon as you wake up, mid-morning and mid-afternoon) and choose the normal or vegan dish: aromatic chicken breast with kale, red onion, tomato sauce, and chili or baked tofu with harissa on spiced cauliflower couscous (vegan dish)

Thursday: 3 green juices

- Breakfast: water + tea or espresso + a cup of green juice;

- Lunch: Sirt food;

- Snack: 1 green juice before dinner

- Dinner: Sirt food

The fourth day of the Sirtfood Diet has arrived, and you are halfway through your journey to a leaner and healthier body. The big change from the previous three days is that you will only drink two juices instead of three and that you will have two solid meals instead of one. This means that on the fourth day and the upcoming ones, you will have two green juices and two solid meals, all delicious and rich in Sirt foods. The inclusion of Medjoul dates in a list of foods that promote weight loss and good health may seem surprising. Especially when you think they contain 66 percent sugar.

Sugar has no stimulating properties towards sirtuins. On the contrary, it has well-known links with obesity, heart disease, and diabetes; in short, just at the antipodes of the objectives, we aim to. But industrially refined and processed sugar is very different from the sugar present in a food that also contains sirtuin-activating polyphenols: the Medjoul dates. Unlike normal sugar, these dates, consumed in moderation, do not increase the level of glucose in the blood.

Today we will also integrate chicory into meals. Like with onion, red chicory is better in this case too, but endive, its close relative, is also a Sirt food. If you are looking for ideas on the use of these salads, combine them with other varieties and season them with olive oil: they will give a pungent flavor to milder leaves.

On the fourth day, you will intake: 2 green Sirt juices, 2 solid meals (normal or vegan)

Drink the juices at different times of the day (for example the first in the morning as soon as you wake up or in the middle of the morning, the second in the middle of the afternoon) and choose the normal or vegan dishes: muesli Sirt, pan-fried salmon fillet with caramelized chicory, rocket salad, and celery leaves or muesli Sirt and Tuscan stewed beans (vegan dish)

Friday: 2 green juices

• Breakfast: water + tea or espresso + a cup of green juice

•   Lunch: Sirt food

•   Snack: a green juice before dinner;

•   Dinner: Sirt food

You have reached the fifth day, and the time has come to add fruits. Due to its high sugar content, fruits have been the subject of bad publicity. This does not apply to berries. Strawberries have a very low sugar content: one teaspoon per 100 grams. They also have an excellent effect on how the body processes simple sugars.

Scientists have found that if we add strawberries to simple sugars, this causes a reduction in insulin demand, and therefore transforms food into a machine that releases energy for a long time. Strawberries are, therefore, a perfect element in diets that will help you lose weight and get back in shape. They are also delicious and extremely versatile, as you will discover in the Sirt version of the fresh and light Middle Eastern tabbouleh.

Miso, made from fermented soy, is a traditional Japanese dish. Miso contains a strong umami taste, a real explosion for the taste buds. In our modern society, we know better monosodium glutamate, artificially created to reproduce the same flavor. Needless to say, it is far preferable to derive that magical umami flavor from traditional and natural food, full of beneficial substances. It is found in the form of a paste in all good supermarkets and healthy food stores and should be present in every kitchen to give a touch of taste to many different dishes.

Since umami flavors enhance each other, miso is perfectly associated with other tasty/umami foods, especially when it comes to cooked proteins, as you will discover today in the very tasty, fast and easy dishes you will eat.

On the fifth day, you will intake 2 green Sirt juices and 2 solid meals (normal or vegan).

Drink the juices at different times of the day (for example the first in the morning as soon as you wake up or in the middle of the morning, the second in the middle of the afternoon) and choose the normal or vegan dishes: buckwheat Tabbouleh with strawberries, baked cod marinated in miso with sautéed vegetables and sesame or buckwheat and strawberry Tabbouleh (vegan dish) and kale (vegan dish).

Saturday: 2 green juices

- Breakfast: water + tea or espresso + a cup of green juice

- Lunch: Sirt food

- Snack: a green juice before dinner;

- Dinner: Sirt food

There are no Sirt foods better than olive oil and red wine. Virgin olive oil is obtained from the fruit only by mechanical means, in conditions that do not deteriorate it, so that you can be sure of its quality and polyphenol content. "Extra virgin" oil is that of the first pressing ("virgin" is the result of the second) and therefore has more flavor and better quality: this is what we strongly recommend you to use when cooking.

No Sirt menu would be complete without red wine, one of the cornerstones of the diet. It contains the activators of resveratrol and piceatannol sirtuins, which probably explain the longevity and slenderness associated with the traditional French way of life, and which are at the origin of the enthusiasm unleashed by Sirt foods.

Of course, wine contains alcohol, so it should be consumed in moderation. Fortunately, resveratrol can withstand heat well, and therefore can be used in the kitchen. Pinot Noir is many people's favorite grape variety because it contains much more resveratrol than most of the others.

On the sixth day, you will assume 2 green Sirt juices and 2 solid meals (normal or vegan).

Drink the juices at different times of the day (for example, the first in the morning as soon as you wake up or in the middle of the morning, the second in the middle of the afternoon) and choose the normal or vegan dishes: Super Sirt salad and grilled beef fillet with red wine sauce, onion rings, garlic curly kale and roasted potatoes with aromatic herbs or

Super lentil Sirt salad (vegan dish) and mole sauce of red beans with roasted potato (vegan dish).

Sunday: 2 green juices

- Breakfast: a bowl of Sirt Muesli + a cup of green juice

- Lunch: Sirt food

- Snack: a cup of green juice;

- Dinner: Sirt food

The seventh day is the last of phase 1 of the diet. Instead of considering it as an end, see it as a beginning, because you are about to embark on a new life, in which Sirt foods will play a central role in your nutrition. Today's menu is a perfect example of how easy it is to integrate them in abundance into your daily diet. Just take your favorite dishes and, with a pinch of creativity, you will turn them into a Sirt banquet.

Walnuts are excellent Sirt food because they contradict current opinions. They have high fat content and many calories, yet it has been shown that they contribute to reducing weight and metabolic diseases, all thanks to the activation of sirtuins. They are also a versatile ingredient, excellent in baked dishes, in salads and as a snack, alone.

Pesto is becoming an irreplaceable ingredient in the kitchen because it is tasty and allows you to give personality to even the simplest dishes. The traditional one is made with basil and pine nuts, but you can try an alternative one with parsley and walnuts. The result is delicious and rich in Sirt foods.

We can apply the same reasoning to an easy-to-prepare dish, such as an omelet. The dish has to be the typical recipe appreciated by the whole family, and simple to transform into a Sirt dish with a few little tricks. In our recipe, we use bacon. Why? Simply because it fits perfectly. The Sirtfood Diet tells us what to include, not what to exclude, and this allows us to change our long-term eating habits. After all, isn't that the secret to not getting back the lost pounds and staying healthy?

On the seventh day, you will assume 2 green Sirt juices; 2 solid meals (normal or vegan).

Drink the juices at different times of the day (for example the first in the morning as soon as you wake up or in the middle of the morning, the second in the middle of the afternoon) and choose the normal or vegan dishes: Sirt omelet Sirt and baked aubergine wedges with walnut and parsley pesto and tomato salad (vegan dish).

During the second phase, there are no calorie restrictions but indications on which Sirt foods must be eaten to consolidate weight loss and not run the risk of getting the lost kilograms back.

Phase 2: maintenance

Congratulations! You have finished the first "hard core" week. The second phase is the easier and is the actual incorporation of sirtuin-filled food selections to your everyday diet or meals. You can call this the "maintenance stage".

By doing so, your body will undergo the fat-burning stage and muscle gain plus a boost on your immune system and overall health.

For this phase, you can now have 3 balanced SirtFood-filled meals each day plus 1 green juice a day.

There is no "dieting", but more on choosing healthier alternatives with adding SirtFood in each meal as much as possible.

I will be providing some recipes for tasty dishes with SirtFood inclusion to further give you an idea on how exciting and healthy this diet journey is.

Now you move back up to a regular calorie intake with the aim to keep your weight loss steady and your Sirtfood intake high. You should have experienced some degree of weight loss by now but you should also feel trimmer and re-invigorated.

Phase 2 lasts for 14 days. During this time you eat 3 sirtfood rich meals, 1 sirtfood green juice and up to 2 optional Sirtfood bite snacks. Strict calorie counting is actively discouraged – if you follow the recommendations and eat balanced meals of reasonable portions, you shouldn't feel hungry or be consuming too much.

You should consume the same beverages you were drinking in phase 1, with the slight change that you are welcome to enjoy the occasional glass of red wine (although don't drink more than 3 per week).

Chapter 6   After The Diet

So, what happens next after Phase 2 of the Sirtfood Diet?

You may repeat the two phases as often as you would like to meet your weight loss goals. Even if you have achieved it, the creators of the diet suggest adopting sirtfoods for your day-to-day needs because they have designed this diet as an alternative way of living.

This means that after the first three weeks, you are encouraged to keep having meals and green juices that are rich in sirtfoods. Other than this, here are some more things that you can do to get more and continue reaping the benefits of sirtfoods for your health:

- Resume your workout routines.

Since your calorie limit for the first couple of weeks into the diet, it is best to either lessen or stop working out while your body gets used to its new condition. No two persons are exactly alike, so the best thing you can do to know when you can start exercising like you usually do it by paying closer attention to your body.

To be on the safer side of things, most followers opt to resume their regular workout schedule after clearing phase 2 of the diet. By then, you would feel more energized, and more capable of completing your usual exercise sets.

Take note that even though a sirtfood diet does not require you to exercise to unlock its benefits, it would still be best for the overall wellness of your body and mind to remain fit and active every day.

- Try out sirtfood smoothies with protein powder.

If you decide to start exercising again, you should add smoothies that contain lots of sirtfoods and protein powder to help you reduce the soreness of your muscles, and keep you well energized throughout and after your workout.

Recipes for fun and tasty sirtfood smoothies can easily be found in blogs and recipe books dedicated to the Sirtfood Diet. If you are pretty confident with your skills in the kitchen, then feel free to experiment with the recommended ingredients, and discover the perfect smoothie combinations for your taste buds.

- Invite your family and friends to try out the diet.

One of the best ways to maintain your healthier diet is by getting the people around you involved in it as well. Studies show that the kind of company you keep can have a huge influence on your lifestyle, including what and how you eat.

Ideally, you can try convincing them by showing the positive effects that the Sirtfood Diet has had on you. Let them also read this guide so that they will have a better idea of what it is, what it can do for them, and how they should go about it.

Consider adopting the principles of the Sirtfood Diet as part of your way of life. It is just not a one-time, quick-fix meal plan, and you cannot go wrong by adding more sirtfoods into your day-to-day diet.

Chapter 7   Sirtfood Diet And Exercise

Joining Exercise with The Sirtfood Diet sirtfood diet and exercise

With 52% of Americans admitting that they think that its simpler to do their charges than to see how to eat steadily, it's fundamental to present a type of eating that turns into a lifestyle as opposed to a coincidental prevailing fashion diet. For a few of us it may not be that difficult to get thinner or hold a solid weight, however the Sirtfood diet can help the individuals who are battling. Be that as it may, shouldn't something be said about joining the Sirtfood diet with work out, is it fitting to stay away from practice totally or present it once you have begun the diet?

The Sirt Diet Principles

With an expected 650 million hefty grown-ups internationally, it's critical to discover smart dieting and exercise systems that are feasible, don't deny you of all that you appreciate, and don't expect you to practice all week. The Sirtfood diet does only that. The thought is that sure nourishments will dynamic the 'thin quality' pathways which are normally actuated by fasting and exercise. Fortunately certain nourishment and drink, including dull chocolate and red wine, contain synthetic substances called polyphenols that enact the qualities that copy the impacts of activity and fasting.

Exercise during the initial barely any weeks

During the main week or two of the diet where your calorie admission is diminished, it is reasonable to stop or lessen practice while your body adjusts to less calories. Tune in to your body and if you feel exhausted or have less vitality than expected, don't work out. Rather guarantee that you stay concentrated on the rules that apply to a solid lifestyle, for example, including satisfactory day by day levels of fiber, protein and products of the soil.

When the diet turns into a lifestyle

When you do practice it's critical to devour protein in a perfect world an hour after your workout. Protein fixes muscles after exercise, lessens irritation and can help recuperation. There are an assortment of plans which incorporate protein which will be ideal for post-practice utilization, for example, the sirt stew con carne or the turmeric chicken and kale serving of mixed greens. If you need something lighter you could attempt the sirt blueberry smoothie and include some protein powder for included advantage. The kind of wellness you do will be down to you, however workouts at home will permit you to pick when to work out, the sorts of activities that suit you and are short and helpful.

The Sirtfood diet is incredible approach to change your dietary patterns, shed pounds and feel more advantageous. The underlying not many weeks may challenge you yet it's imperative to check which nourishments are ideal to eat and which scrumptious plans suit you. Be benevolent to yourself in the initial barely any weeks while your body adjusts and take practice simple if you decide to do it by any stretch of the imagination. If you are as of now somebody who moderates or extreme exercise then it might be that you can carry on as ordinary, or deal with your wellness as per the adjustment in diet. Similarly as with any diet and exercise changes, it's about the individual and how far you can propel yourself.

Minerals and nutrients for which ladies may require supplements incorporate calcium, iron, Vitamins B6, B12 and D. Men, be that as it may, need to focus on fiber, magnesium, Vitamins B9, C and E.

That reason applies to weight loss diets also. People's nourishment necessities sway which weight loss diets are increasingly compelling for each sex.

If you're similar to the vast majority, you've seen an astounding number of weight loss projects and patterns go back and forth; practically every one of them have their benefits and practically every one of them work — incidentally. Weight the executives and therapeutic experts fight collectively that the deep rooted, proven blend of good sustenance and ordinary exercise is the most ideal approach to adequately shed pounds and keep it off.

The Sirtfood Diet: For Women Only?

When the Sirtfood Diet started slanting, ladies all around hurled a murmur of delight. At last! Not just authorization to enjoy the two most pleasurable edibles on the planet — dull chocolate and red wine — yet support and justification! Then again, men may survey the diet and ask, "Where's the meat?"

"Sirtfood" is nourishment high in sirtuin proteins. The super-nourishments that are remembered for the Sirtfood Diet include:

•Apples

- Blueberries

- Buckwheat

- Capers

- Citrus natural products

- Dark chocolate in any event 85% cacao

- Extra-virgin olive oil

- Green tea

- Kale

- Medjool dates

- Parsley

- Red onions

- Red wine

- Rocket

- Turmeric

- Walnuts

It's accounted for that a diet high in these "super-nourishments" will:

- Burn fat

- Increase bulk

- Regulate digestion

The Diet — Phase 1

For three days, limit calories to 1,000/day and limit nourishments to three sirtfood green juices or smoothies (any blend of celery, kale, parsley) and 1 dinner/day sirtfood-rich (turkey/chicken with escapades, parsley, sage). Starting on day 4 through day seven, increment calories to 1,500/day with 2 sirtfood green juices or smoothies and 2 sirtfood-rich dinners/day.

The Diet — Phase 2

For the accompanying two weeks, you'll consider a to be weight loss as you eat 3 sirtfood-rich dinners every day and one sirtfood green juice or smoothie.

How Is This Diet Different?

The Sirtfood Diet is different from different diets you've attempted in light of the fact that you won't see emotional weight loss. Defenders state you'll see strong weight loss that is consistent and offers the guarantee of long haul benefits. Similarly as with any dietary shift, you ought to counsel with your GP or restorative specialist before starting the Sirtfood Diet.

You'll discover plans in abundance on the web or can make your own utilizing lean meat, foods grown from the ground. Sides can remember seared red onion for olive oil, buckwheat and steamed kale.

At Holmes Place, we accept people's nourishment is critical to in general health. Our main goal is to urge and move individuals to diet, practice and create pressure decrease abilities, as per what is refreshing for every person. Make certain to investigate our site for extraordinary formula thoughts.

Sirtfood for all

Numerous wellbeing cognizant individuals are focused on a specific style of eating, with any semblance of discontinuous fasting with the 5:2 and different weight control plans, low-carb, paleo, including the Dukan Diet, and without gluten eats less being particularly mainstream. While they don't work for a few, many vouches for them.

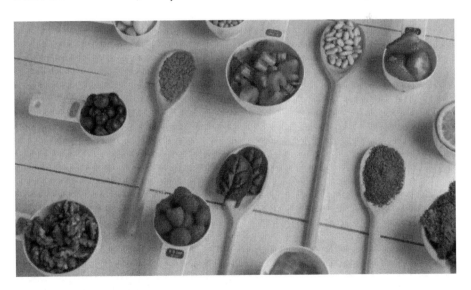

Be that as it may, how do Sirtfoods fit in with these different weight control plans?

1. Sirtfoods are good with all other dietary methodologies as well as can effectively improve their advantages.

2. Low-carb counts calories that need plant-based nourishments can be drastically enlarged by the consideration of Sirtfoods.

3. Sirtfoods are the regular paleo nourishments, containing the sirtuin-enacting polyphenols that people would have developed eating and receiving the rewards from over an exceptionally extensive stretch of time.

4. The best 20 Sirtfoods are normally without gluten making them a genuine advantage for anybody following a sans gluten diet.

Chapter 8   Questions And Answers

You have likely found answers to most of your questions about the Sirt diet throughout the pages of this book. However, I will seek to answer any remaining questions you might have so that you can begin your journey to success with ease and confidence.

Can Children Eat Sirtfoods?

There are powerful sirtfoods, most of which are safe for children. Obviously, children should avoid wine, coffee, and other highly caffeinated foods, such as matcha. On the other hand, children can enjoy sirtuin-rich foods such as cabbage, eggplant, blueberries, and dates with their regular balanced diet.

Yet, while children can enjoy most sirtuin-rich foods, that is not the same as to say that they can practice the Sirt diet. This diet plan is not designed for children, and it does not fit the needs of their growing bodies. Practicing this diet plan could not only negatively affect them physically, but it could damage their mental health for years to come. Anyone can develop an eating disorder, but it is especially true for children. If you want your child to eat well, ensure they eat a wide range of foods, as recommended by their doctor, and you can simply include an abundance of sirtuin-rich foods into what they are already eating. Leave the focus on eating healthfully and not losing weight. Even if your child's doctor does want them to lose weight, you don't need to make the child aware of this fact. You can help guide them along with a healthy lifestyle, teaching them how to eat well and stay active through sports and play, and the weight will come off naturally without placing an unneeded burden on their small shoulders.

For similar reasons, you can include sirtfoods in a balanced diet while pregnant, but you should avoid practicing the Sirt diet when you are pregnant. It doesn't contain the nutrition requirements for either a pregnant woman or a growing baby. Save the diet for after you have delivered a healthy baby, and both you and your child will be healthy and happy.

Can I Exercise During Phase One?

If you use exercise during either phase one or two, you can increase weight loss and health benefits. While you shouldn't work at pushing the limits during phase one, you can continue your normal workout routine and physical activity. It is important to stay within your active comfort zone during this time, as physical exertion more than you are accustomed to will be especially difficult while you are restricting your calories. It will not only wear you out, but it can also make you dizzy, more prone to injury, and physically and mentally exhausted. This is a common symptom whenever a person pushes their limits while restricting calories, but it is something you should avoid.

If you are used to doing yoga and a spin class a few times a week, keep it up! If you are used to running a few miles a day, have at it! Do what you and your body are comfortable with, and as your doctor advises, and you should be fine.

I'm Already Thin. Can I Still Follow The Diet?

Whether or not you can follow the first phase of the Sirt diet will depend just how thin you already are. While a person who is overweight or well within a healthy weight can practice the first phase, nobody who is clinically underweight should. You can know whether or not you are underweight by calculating your Body Mass Index, or BMI. You can find many BMI calculators online, and if yours is at nineteen points or below, you should avoid the first phase. It is always a good idea to ask your doctor both if it is safe for you to lose weight, and if the Sirt diet is safe for your individual condition. While the Sirt diet may generally be safe, for people with certain illnesses, it may not be the case.

While it is understandable to desire to be even more thin, even if you already are thin, pushing yourself past the point of being underweight is incredibly unhealthy, both physically and mentally. This fits into the category of disordered eating and can cause you a lot of harm.

Some of the side effects of pushing your body to extreme weight loss include bone loss and osteoporosis, lowered immune system, fertility problems, and an increased risk of disease. If you want to benefit from the health of the Sirt diet and are underweight, instead consume, however many calories, your doctor recommends, along with plenty of sirtfoods. This will ensure you maintain a healthy weight while also receiving the benefits that sirtuins have to offer.

If you are thin, but still at a BMI of twenty to twenty-five, then you should be safe beginning the Sirt diet, unless otherwise instructed by your doctor.

Can You Eat Meat and Dairy On The Sirtfood Diet?

In many recipes, we choose to use sirtfood sources of protein, such as soy, walnuts, and buckwheat. However, this does not mean that you aren't allowed to enjoy meat on the Sirt diet. Sure, it's easy to enjoy a vegan or vegetarian Sirt diet, but if you love your sources of meat, then you don't have to give them up. Protein is an essential aspect of the Sirt diet to preserve muscle tone, and whether you consume only plant-based proteins or a mixture of plant and animal-based proteins is completely up to you. And, just as you can enjoy meat, you can also enjoy moderate consumption of dairy.

Some meats can actually help you better utilize the sirtfoods you eat. This is because the amino acid leucine is able to enhance the effect of sirtfoods. You can find this amino acid in chicken, beef, pork, fish, eggs, dairy, and tofu.

Can I Drink Red Wine during Phase One?

As your calories will be so limited during the first phase, it is not recommended to drink alcohol during this phase. However, you can enjoy it in moderation during phase two and the maintenance phase.

Chapter 9   Recipes

Matcha Green Juice

Preparation time: 10 minutes

Cooking time: 0 minutes

Servings: 2

Ingredients:

5 ounces fresh kale

2 ounces fresh arugula

¼ cup fresh parsley

4 celery stalks

1 green apple, cored and chopped

1 (1-inch) piece fresh ginger, peeled

1 lemon, peeled

½ teaspoon matcha green tea

Directions:

Add all ingredients into a juicer and extract the juice according to the manufacturer's method.

Pour into 2 glasses and serve immediately.

Nutrition:

Calories 113

Fat 0.6 g

Carbs 26.71 g

Protein 3.8 g

Celery Juice

Preparation time: 10 minutes

Cooking time: 0 minutes

Servings: 2

Ingredients:

8 celery stalks with leaves

2 tablespoons fresh ginger, peeled

1 lemon, peeled

½ cup filtered water

Pinch of salt

Directions:

Place all the ingredients in a blender and pulse until well combined.

Through a fine mesh strainer, strain the juice and transfer into 2 glasses.

Serve immediately.

Nutrition:

Calories 32

Fat 0.5 g

Carbs 6.5 g

Protein 1 g

Kale & Orange Juice

Preparation time: 10 minutes

Cooking time: 0 minutes

Servings: 2

Ingredients:

5 large oranges, peeled and sectioned

2 bunches fresh kale

Directions:

Add all ingredients into a juicer and extract the juice according to the manufacturer's method.

Pour into 2 glasses and serve immediately.

Nutrition:

Calories 315

Fat 0.6 g

Carbs 75.1 g

Protein 10.3 g

Apple & Cucumber Juice

Preparation time: 10 minutes

Cooking time: 0 minutes

Servings: 2

Ingredients:

3 large apples, cored and sliced

2 large cucumbers, sliced

4 celery stalks

1 (1-inch) piece fresh ginger, peeled

1 lemon, peeled

Directions:

Add all ingredients into a juicer and extract the juice according to the manufacturer's method.

Pour into 2 glasses and serve immediately.

Nutrition:

Calories 230

Fat 1.1 g

Carbs 59.5 g

Protein 3.3 g

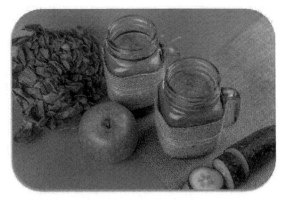

Lemony Green Juice

Preparation time: 10 minutes

Cooking time: 0 minutes

Servings: 2

Ingredients:

2 large green apples, cored and sliced

4 cups fresh kale leaves

4 tablespoons fresh parsley leaves

1 tablespoon fresh ginger, peeled

1 lemon, peeled

½ cup filtered water

Pinch of salt

Directions:

Place all the ingredients in a blender and pulse until well combined.

Through a fine mesh strainer, strain the juice and transfer into 2 glasses.

Serve immediately.

Nutrition:

Calories 196

Fat 0.6 g

Carbs 47.9 g

Protein 5.2 g

Kale Scramble

Preparation time: 10 minutes

Cooking time: 6 minutes

Servings: 2

Ingredients:

4 eggs

1/8 teaspoon ground turmeric

Salt and ground black pepper, to taste

1 tablespoon water

2 teaspoons olive oil

1 cup fresh kale, tough ribs removed and chopped

Directions:

In a bowl, add the eggs, turmeric, salt, black pepper, and water and with a whisk, beat until foamy.

In a wok, heat the oil over medium heat.

Add the egg mixture and stir to combine.

Immediately, reduce the heat to medium-low and cook for about 1–2 minutes, stirring frequently.

Stir in the kale and cook for about 3–4 minutes, stirring frequently.

Remove from the heat and serve immediately.

Nutrition:

Calories 183

Fat 13.4 g

Carbs 4.3 g

Protein 12.1 g

Buckwheat Porridge

Preparation time: 10 minutes

Cooking time: 15 minutes

Servings: 2

Ingredients

1 cup buckwheat, rinsed

1 cup unsweetened almond milk

1 cup water

½ teaspoon ground cinnamon

½ teaspoon vanilla extract

1–2 tablespoons raw honey

¼ cup fresh blueberries

Directions:

In a pan, add all the ingredients (except honey and blueberries) over medium-high heat and bring to a boil.

Now, reduce the heat to low and simmer, covered for about 10 minutes.

Stir in the honey and remove from the heat.

Set aside, covered, for about 5 minutes.

With a fork, fluff the mixture, and transfer into serving bowls.

Top with blueberries and serve.

Nutrition:

Calories 358

Fat 4.7 g

Carbs 3.7 g

Protein 12 g

Chocolate Granola

Preparation time: 10 minutes

Cooking time: 38 minutes

Servings: 8

Ingredients

¼ cup cacao powder

¼ cup maple syrup

2 tablespoons coconut oil, melted

½ teaspoon vanilla extract

1/8 teaspoon salt

2 cups gluten-free rolled oats

¼ cup unsweetened coconut flakes

2 tablespoons chia seeds

2 tablespoons unsweetened dark chocolate, chopped finely

Directions:

Preheat your oven to 300°F and line a medium baking sheet with parchment paper.

In a medium pan, add the cacao powder, maple syrup, coconut oil, vanilla extract, and salt, and mix well.

Now, place pan over medium heat and cook for about 2–3 minutes, or until thick and syrupy, stirring continuously.

Remove from the heat and set aside.

In a large bowl, add the oats, coconut, and chia seeds, and mix well.

Add the syrup mixture and mix until well combined.

Transfer the granola mixture onto a prepared baking sheet and spread in an even layer.

Bake for about 35 minutes.

Remove from the oven and set aside for about 1 hour.

Add the chocolate pieces and stir to combine.

Serve immediately.

Nutrition:

Calories 193

Fat 9.1 g

Carbs 26.1 g

Protein 5 g

Blueberry Muffins

Preparation time: 15 minutes

Cooking time: 20 minutes

Servings: 8

Ingredients

1 cup buckwheat flour

¼ cup arrowroot starch

1½ teaspoons baking powder

¼ teaspoon sea salt

2 eggs

½ cup unsweetened almond milk

2–3 tablespoons maple syrup

2 tablespoons coconut oil, melted

1 cup fresh blueberries

Directions:

Preheat your oven to 350°F and line 8 cups of a muffin tin.

In a bowl, place the buckwheat flour, arrowroot starch, baking powder, and salt, and mix well.

In a separate bowl, place the eggs, almond milk, maple syrup, and coconut oil, and beat until well combined.

Now, place the flour mixture and mix until just combined.

Gently, fold in the blueberries.

Transfer the mixture into prepared muffin cups evenly.

Bake for about 25 minutes or until a toothpick inserted in the center comes out clean.

Remove the muffin tin from oven and place onto a wire rack to cool for about 10 minutes.

Carefully invert the muffins onto the wire rack to cool completely before serving.

Nutrition:

Calories 136

Fat 5.3 g

Carbs 20.7 g

Protein 3.5 g

Chocolate Waffles

Preparation time: 15 minutes

Cooking time: 24 minutes

Servings: 8

Ingredients

2 cups unsweetened almond milk

1 tablespoon fresh lemon juice

1 cup buckwheat flour

½ cup cacao powder

¼ cup flaxseed meal

1 teaspoon baking soda

1 teaspoon baking powder

¼ teaspoons kosher salt

2 large eggs

½ cup coconut oil, melted

¼ cup dark brown sugar

2 teaspoons vanilla extract

2 ounces unsweetened dark chocolate, chopped roughly

Directions:

In a bowl, add the almond milk and lemon juice and mix well.

Set aside for about 10 minutes.

In a bowl, place buckwheat flour, cacao powder, flaxseed meal, baking soda, baking powder, and salt, and mix well.

In the bowl of almond milk mixture, place the eggs, coconut oil, brown sugar, and vanilla extract, and beat until smooth.

Now, place the flour mixture and beat until smooth.

Gently, fold in the chocolate pieces.

Preheat the waffle iron and then grease it.

Place the desired amount of the mixture into the preheated waffle iron and cook for about 3 minutes, or until golden-brown.

Repeat with the remaining mixture.

Nutrition:

Calories 295

Fat 22.1 g

Carbs 1.5 g

Protein 6.3 g

Salmon & Kale Omelet

Preparation time: 10 minutes

Cooking time: 7 minutes

Servings: 4

Ingredients

6 eggs

2 tablespoons unsweetened almond milk

Salt and ground black pepper, to taste

2 tablespoons olive oil

4 ounces smoked salmon, cut into bite-sized chunks

2 cup fresh kale, tough ribs removed and chopped finely

4 scallions, chopped finely

Directions:

In a bowl, place the eggs, coconut milk, salt, and black pepper, and beat well. Set aside.

In a non-stick wok, heat the oil over medium heat.

Place the egg mixture evenly and cook for about 30 seconds, without stirring.

Place the salmon kale and scallions on top of egg mixture evenly.

Now, reduce heat to low.

With the lid, cover the wok and cook for about 4–5 minutes, or until omelet is done completely.

Uncover the wok and cook for about 1 minute.

Carefully, transfer the omelet onto a serving plate and serve.

Nutrition:

Calories 210

Fat 14.9 g

Carbs 5.2 g

Protein 14.8 g

Moroccan Spiced Eggs

Preparation time: 1 hour

Cooking time: 50 minutes

Servings: 2

Ingredients:

1 tsp olive oil

One shallot, stripped and finely hacked

One red (chime) pepper, deseeded and finely hacked

One garlic clove, stripped and finely hacked

One courgette (zucchini), stripped and finely hacked

1 tbsp tomato puree (glue)

½ tsp gentle stew powder

¼ tsp ground cinnamon

¼ tsp ground cumin

½ tsp salt

One × 400g (14oz) can hacked tomatoes

1 x 400g (14oz) may chickpeas in water

a little bunch of level leaf parsley (10g (1/3oz)), cleaved

Four medium eggs at room temperature

Directions:

Heat the oil in a pan, include the shallot and red (ringer) pepper and fry delicately for 5 minutes. At that point include the garlic and courgette (zucchini) and cook for one more moment or two. Include the tomato puree (glue), flavours and salt and mix through.

Add the cleaved tomatoes and chickpeas (dousing alcohol and all) and increment the warmth to medium. With the top of the dish, stew the sauce for 30 minutes – ensure it is delicately rising all through and permit it to lessen in volume by around 33%.

Remove from the warmth and mix in the cleaved parsley.

Preheat the grill to 200C/180C fan/350F.

When you are prepared to cook the eggs, bring the tomato sauce up to a delicate stew and move to a little broiler confirmation dish.

Crack the eggs on the dish and lower them delicately into the stew. Spread with thwart and prepare in the grill for 10-15 minutes. Serve the blend in unique dishes with the eggs coasting on the top.

Nutrition:

Calories: 116 kcal

Protein: 6.97 g

Fat: 5.22 g

Carbohydrates: 13.14 g

Chilaquiles with Gochujang

Preparation time: 30 minutes

Cooking time: 20 minutes

Servings: 2

Ingredients:

One dried ancho chile

2 cups of water

1 cup squashed tomatoes

Two cloves of garlic

One teaspoon genuine salt

1/2 tablespoons gochujang

5 to 6 cups tortilla chips

Three enormous eggs

One tablespoon olive oil

Directions:

Get the water to heat a pot. I cheated marginally and heated the water in an electric pot and emptied it into the pan. There's no sound unrivalled strategy here. Add the anchor Chile to the bubbled water and drench for 15 minutes to give it an opportunity to stout up.

When completed, use tongs or a spoon to extricate Chile. Make sure to spare the water for the sauce! Nonetheless, on the off chance that you incidentally dump the water, it's not the apocalypse.

Mix the doused Chile, 1 cup of saved high temp water, squashed tomatoes, garlic, salt and gochujang until smooth.

Empty sauce into a large dish and warmth over medium warmth for 4 to 5 minutes. Mood killer the heat and include the tortilla chips. Mix the chips to cover with the sauce. In a different skillet, shower a teaspoon of oil and fry an egg on top, until the whites have settled. Plate the egg and cook the remainder of the eggs. If you are phenomenal at performing various tasks, you can likely sear the eggs while you heat the red sauce. I am not precisely so capable.

Top the chips with the seared eggs, cotija, hacked cilantro, jalapeños, onions and avocado. Serve right away.

Nutrition:

Calories: 484 kcal

Protein: 14.55 g

Fat: 18.62 g

Carbohydrates: 64.04 g

Twice Baked Breakfast Potatoes

Preparation time: 1 hour 10 minutes

Cooking time: 1 hour

Servings: 2

Ingredients:

2 medium reddish brown potatoes, cleaned and pricked with a fork everywhere

2 tablespoons unsalted spread

3 tablespoons overwhelming cream

4 rashers cooked bacon

4 huge eggs

½ cup destroyed cheddar

Daintily cut chives

Salt and pepper to taste

Directions:

Preheat grill to 400°F.

Spot potatoes straightforwardly on stove rack in the focal point of the grill and prepare for 30 to 45 min.

Evacuate and permit potatoes to cool for around 15 minutes.

Cut every potato down the middle longwise and burrow every half out, scooping the potato substance into a blending bowl.

Gather margarine and cream to the potato and pound into a single unit until smooth — season with salt and pepper and mix.

Spread a portion of the potato blend into the base of each emptied potato skin and sprinkle with one tablespoon cheddar (you may make them remain pounded potato left to snack on).

Add one rasher bacon to every half and top with a raw egg.

Spot potatoes onto a heating sheet and come back to the appliance.

Lower broiler temperature to 375°F and heat potatoes until egg whites simply set and yolks are as yet runny.

Top every potato with a sprinkle of the rest of the cheddar, season with salt and pepper and finish with cut chives.

Nutrition:

Calories: 647 kcal

Protein: 30.46 g

Fat: 55.79 g

Carbohydrates: 7.45 g

Sirt Muesli

Preparation time: 30 minutes

Cooking time: 0 minutes

Servings: 2

Ingredients:

20g buckwheat drops

10g buckwheat puffs

15g coconut drops or dried up coconut

40g Medjool dates, hollowed and slashed

15g pecans, slashed

10g cocoa nibs

100g strawberries, hulled and slashed

100g plain Greek yoghurt (or vegetarian elective, for example, soya or coconut yoghurt)

Directions:

Blend the entirety of the above fixings (forget about the strawberries and yoghurt if not serving straight away).

Nutrition:

Calories: 334 kcal

Protein: 4.39 g

Fat: 22.58 g

Carbohydrates: 34.35 g

Mushroom Scramble Eggs

Preparation time: 45 minutes

Cooking time: 10 minutes

Servings: 2

Ingredients:

2 eggs

1 tsp ground turmeric

1 tsp mellow curry powder

20g kale, generally slashed

1 tsp additional virgin olive oil

½ superior bean stew, daintily cut

bunch of catch mushrooms, meagerly cut

5g parsley, finely slashed

optional Add a seed blend as a topper and some Rooster Sauce for enhance

Directions:

Blend the turmeric and curry powder and include a little water until you have accomplished a light glue.

Steam the kale for 2–3 minutes.

Warmth the oil in a skillet over medium heat and fry the bean stew and mushrooms for 2–3 minutes until they have begun to darker and mollify.

Include the eggs and flavour glue and cook over a medium warmth at that point add the kale and keep on cooking over medium heat for a further moment. At long last, include the parsley, blend well and serve.

Nutrition:

Calories: 158 kcal

Protein: 9.96 g

Fat: 10.93 g

Carbohydrates: 5.04 g

Smoked Salmon Omelets

Preparation time: 45 minutes

Cooking time: 15 minutes

Servings: 2

Ingredients:

2 Medium eggs

100 g Smoked salmon, cut

1/2 tsp Capers

10 g Rocket, slashed

1 tsp Parsley, slashed

1 tsp extra virgin olive oil

Directions:

Split the eggs into a bowl and whisk well. Include the salmon, tricks, rocket and parsley.

Warmth the olive oil in a non-stick skillet until hot yet not smoking. Include the egg blend and, utilizing a spatula or fish cut, move the mixture around the dish until it is even. Diminish the warmth and let the omelet cook through. Slide the spatula around the edges and move up or crease the omelet fifty-fifty to serve.

Nutrition:

Calories: 148 kcal

Protein: 15.87 g

Fat: 8.73 g

Carbohydrates: 0.36 g

Date and Walnut Porridge

Preparation time: 55 minutes

Cooking time: 30 minutes

Servings: 2

Ingredients:

200 ml Milk or without dairy elective

1 Medjool date, hacked

35 g Buckwheat chips

1 tsp. Pecan spread or four cleaved pecan parts

50 g Strawberries, hulled

Directions:

Spot the milk and time in a dish, heat tenderly, at that point include the buckwheat chips and cook until the porridge is your ideal consistency.

Mix in the pecan margarine or pecans, top with the strawberries and serve.

Nutrition:

Calories: 66 kcal

Protein: 1.08 g

Fat: 1.07 g

Carbohydrates: 14.56 g

Shakshuka

Preparation time: 55 minutes

Cooking time: 30 minutes

Servings: 2

Ingredients:

1 tsp extra virgin olive oil

40g Red onion, finely hacked

1 Garlic clove, finely hacked

30g Celery, finely hacked

1 Bird's eye stew, finely hacked

1 tsp ground cumin

1 tsp ground turmeric

1 tsp Paprika

400g Tinned hacked tomatoes

30g Kale stems expelled and generally hacked

1 tbsp Chopped parsley

2 Medium eggs

Directions:

Heat a little, profound sided skillet over medium-low warmth. Include the oil and fry the onion, garlic, celery, stew and flavours for 1–2 minutes.

Add the tomatoes, at that point, leave the sauce to stew tenderly for 20 minutes, mixing incidentally.

Add the kale and cook for a more 5 minutes. If you realize the sauce is getting excessively thick, just include a little water. At the point when your sauce has a pleasant creamy consistency, mix in the parsley.

Make two small wells in the sauce and split each egg into them. Decrease the warmth to its most minimal setting and spread the container with a cover or foil. Put the eggs to cook for 10–12 minutes, so, all in all, the whites ought to be firm while the yolks are as yet runny. Cook a further 3–4 minutes if you lean toward the eggs to be firm. Serve promptly – in a perfect world directly from the skillet.

Nutrition:

Calories: 135 kcal

Protein: 9.41 g

Fat: 6.16 g

Carbohydrates: 12.65 g

Moroccan Spiced Eggs

Preparation time: 1 hour 10 minutes

Cooking time: 45 minutes

Servings: 2

Ingredients:

1 tsp olive oil

One shallot, stripped and finely hacked

One red (chime) pepper, deseeded and finely hacked

One garlic clove, stripped and finely hacked

One courgette (zucchini), stripped and finely hacked

1 tbsp tomato puree (glue)

½ tsp gentle stew powder

¼ tsp ground cinnamon

¼ tsp ground cumin

½ tsp salt

One × 400g (14oz) can hacked tomatoes

1 x 400g (14oz) may chickpeas in water

a little bunch of level leaf parsley (10g (1/3oz)), cleaved

Four medium eggs at room temperature

Directions:

Heat the oil in a pan, include the shallot and red (ringer) pepper and fry delicately for 5 minutes. At that point include the garlic and courgette (zucchini) and cook for one more moment or two. Include the tomato puree (glue), flavours and salt and mix through.

Add the cleaved tomatoes and chickpeas (dousing alcohol and all) and increment the warmth to medium. With the top of the dish, stew the sauce for 30 minutes – ensure it is delicately rising all through and permit it to lessen in volume by around 33%.

Remove from the warmth and mix in the cleaved parsley.

Preheat the grill to 200C/180C fan/350F.

When you are prepared to cook the eggs, bring the tomato sauce up to a delicate stew and move to a little broiler confirmation dish.

Crack the eggs on the dish and lower them delicately into the stew. Spread with thwart and prepare in the grill for 10-15 minutes. Serve the blend in unique dishes with the eggs coasting on the top.

Nutrition:

Calorie: 116 kcal

Protein: 6.97 g

Fat: 5.22 g

Carbohydrates: 13.14 g

Exquisite Turmeric Pancakes with Lemon Yogurt Sauce

Preparation time: 45 minutes

Cooking time: 15 minutes

Servings: 8 hotcakes

Ingredients:

For The Yogurt Sauce

1 cup plain Greek yogurt

1 garlic clove, minced

1 to 2 tablespoons lemon juice (from 1 lemon), to taste

¼ teaspoon ground turmeric

10 crisp mint leaves, minced

2 teaspoons lemon pizzazz (from 1 lemon)

For The Pancakes

2 teaspoons ground turmeric

1½ teaspoons ground cumin

1 teaspoon salt

1 teaspoon ground coriander

½ teaspoon garlic powder

½ teaspoon naturally ground dark pepper

1 head broccoli, cut into florets

3 enormous eggs, gently beaten

2 tablespoons plain unsweetened almond milk

1 cup almond flour

4 teaspoons coconut oil

Directions:

Make the yogurt sauce. Join the yogurt, garlic, lemon juice, turmeric, mint and pizzazz in a bowl. Taste and enjoy with more lemon juice, if possible. Keep in a safe spot or freeze until prepared to serve.

Make the flapjacks. In a little bowl, join the turmeric, cumin, salt, coriander, garlic and pepper.

Spot the broccoli in a nourishment processor, and heartbeat until the florets are separated into little pieces. Move the broccoli to an enormous bowl and include the eggs, almond milk, and almond flour. Mix in the flavor blend and consolidate well.

Heat 1 teaspoon of the coconut oil in a nonstick dish over medium-low heat. Empty ¼ cup player into the skillet. Cook the hotcake until little air pockets start to show up superficially and the base is brilliant darker, 2 to 3 minutes. Flip over and cook the hotcake for 2 to 3 minutes more. To keep warm, move the cooked hotcakes to a stove safe dish and spot in a 200°F oven.

Keep making the staying 3 hotcakes, utilizing the rest of the oil and player.

Nutrition:

Calories: 262 kcal

Protein: 11.68 g

Fat: 19.28 g

Carbohydrates: 12.06 g

Sirt Chili Con Carne

Preparation time: 1 hour 20 minutes

Cooking time: 1 hour 3 minutes

Servings: 4

Ingredients:

1 red onion, finely cleaved

3 garlic cloves, finely cleaved

2 10,000 foot chillies, finely hacked

1 tbsp additional virgin olive oil

1 tbsp ground cumin

1 tbsp ground turmeric

400g lean minced hamburger (5 percent fat)

150ml red wine

1 red pepper, cored, seeds evacuated and cut into reduced down pieces

2 x 400g tins cleaved tomatoes

1 tbsp tomato purée

1 tbsp cocoa powder

150g tinned kidney beans

300ml hamburger stock

5g coriander, cleaved

5g parsley, cleaved

160g buckwheat

Directions:

In a meal, fry the onion, garlic and bean stew in the oil over a medium heat for 2-3 minutes, at that point include the flavors and cook for a moment.

Include the minced hamburger and dark colored over a high heat. Include the red wine and permit it to rise to decrease it considerably.

Include the red pepper, tomatoes, tomato purée, cocoa, kidney beans and stock and leave to stew for 60 minutes.

You may need to add a little water to accomplish a thick, clingy consistency. Just before serving, mix in the hacked herbs.

In the interim, cook the buckwheat as indicated by the bundle guidelines and present with the stew.

Nutrition:

Calories: 346 kcal

Protein: 14.11 g

Fat: 11.37 g

Carbohydrates: 49.25 g

Chickpea, Quinoa and Turmeric Curry Recipe

Preparation time: 1 hour 10 minutes

Cooking time: 1 hour

Servings: 6

Ingredients:

500g new potatoes, split

3 garlic cloves, squashed

3 teaspoons ground turmeric

1 teaspoon ground coriander

1 teaspoon stew drops or powder

1 teaspoon ground ginger

400g container of coconut milk

1 tbsp tomato purée

400g container of slashed tomatoes

Salt and pepper

180g quinoa

400g container of chickpeas, depleted and flushed

150g spinach

Directions:

Spot the potatoes in a dish of cold water and bring to the boil, at that point let them cook for around 25 minutes until you can undoubtedly stick a blade through them. Channel them well.

Spot the potatoes in an enormous skillet and include the garlic, turmeric, coriander, bean stew, ginger, coconut milk, tomato purée and tomatoes. Bring to the boil, season with salt and pepper, at that point include the quinoa with a cup of simply boil water (300ml).

Diminish the heat to a stew, place the top on and permit to cook. Throughout the following 30 minutes, blending at regular intervals or so to ensure nothing adheres to the base. (This is a significant long cooking time, yet this is to what extent quinoa takes to cook in every one of these Ingredients:, as opposed to simply in water.) Halfway through cooking, include the chickpeas. When there are only 5 minutes left, include the spinach and mix it in until it withers. Once the quinoa has cooked and is cushioned, not crunchy, it's prepared.

On the off chance that you like a touch of heat, add a cut red bean stew to the cooking curry simultaneously as different flavors

Nutrition:

Calories: 609 kcal

Protein: 23.04 g

Fat: 22.15 g

Carbohydrates: 85.27 g

Baked Salmon Salad with Creamy Mint Dressing

Preparation time: 55 minutes

Cooking time: 20 minutes

Serving: 1

Ingredients

1 salmon fillet (130g)

40g mixed salad leaves

40g young spinach leaves

2 radishes, trimmed and thinly sliced

5cm piece (50g) cucumber, cut into chunks

2 spring onions, trimmed and sliced

one small handful (10g) parsley, roughly chopped

For the dressing

1 tsp low-fat mayonnaise

1 tbsp natural yoghurt

1 tbsp rice vinegar

2 leaves mint, finely chopped

Salt to taste

Freshly ground black pepper

Directions:

First, preheat your oven to 200°C

(180°C fan/Gas 6).

Now place the salmon fillet on a baking tray. Bake it for 16–18 minutes until cooked. Now remove it from the oven and set aside. The salmon is equally useful to be you used as hot or cold in the salad. If salmon has skin, simply cook skin side down. Remove the salmon from the skin. It slides off easily when cooked.

Now mix the mayonnaise, yoghurt, rice wine vinegar, and the mint leaves. Add salt and pepper.

Leave them to stand for at least 5 minutes. It allows the flavours to develop.

Arrange salad leaves and spinach on a serving plate. Top with the radishes, cucumber, the spring onions and parsley. Now Flake the cooked salmon onto the salad. Finally, drizzle the dressing over.

Nutrition:

Calories: 483 kcal

Protein: 13.82 g

Fat: 33.89 g

Carbohydrates: 34.89 g

Coronation Chicken Salad

Preparation time: 5 minutes

Cooking time: 0 minutes

Servings: 1

Ingredients

75 g Natural yoghurt

Juice of 1/4 of a lemon

1 tsp Coriander, chopped

1 tsp ground turmeric

1/2 tsp Mild curry powder

100 g Cooked chicken breast, cut into bite-sized pieces

6 Walnut halves, finely chopped

1 Medjool date, finely chopped

20 g Red onion, diced

1 Bird's eye chilli

40 g Rocket (for serving)

Directions:

Mix the yoghurt, lemon juice, coriander and the spices. Add all the remaining ingredients now. Serve on a bed of the rocket.

Nutrition:

Calories: 831 kcal

Protein: 27.47 g

Fat: 77.64 g

Carbohydrates: 19.93 g

Baked Potatoes with Spicy Chickpea Stew

Preparation time: 10 minutes

Cooking time: 1 hour

Servings: 4-6

Ingredients

4-6 baking potatoes, pricked all over

2 tablespoons olive oil

2 red onions, finely chopped

4 cloves garlic, grated or crushed

2cm ginger, grated

½ -2 teaspoons chilli flakes (depending on how hot you like things)

2 tablespoons cumin seeds

2 tablespoons turmeric

Splash of water

2 x 400g tins chopped tomatoes

2 tablespoons unsweetened cocoa powder (or cacao)

2 x 400g tins chickpeas (or kidney beans if you prefer) including the chickpea water DON'T DRAIN!!

2 yellow peppers (or whatever colour you prefer!), chopped into bite size pieces

2 tablespoons parsley plus extra for garnish

Salt and pepper to taste (optional)

Side salad

Directions:

Preheat the oven to 200C.

Meanwhile prepare all the other ingredients.

When the oven is hot enough, then put your baking potatoes in the oven. Cook for 1 hour.

Once the potatoes are in the oven, then place the olive oil and chopped red onion in a large wide saucepan. Cook it gently, with the lid on for 5 minutes. Continue cooking until the onions are soft but not brown.

Remove the lid. Add the garlic, ginger, cumin and chilli. Now cook for a minute on low heat. Then add the turmeric and a tiny splash of water and cook for one minute. Take care that pan does get too dry.

Now add in the tomatoes, cocoa powder (or cacao), chickpeas (also include the chickpea water). Also, add yellow pepper and bring to boil. Simmer on a low heat for about 45 minutes. Hence the sauce is thick (but don't let it burn!).

The stew should be cooked roughly at the same time as the potatoes.

Finally, stir in the two tablespoons of parsley, and some salt and pepper if you wish. Finally, serve the stew on top of the baked potatoes.

Nutrition:

Calories: 322 kcal

Protein: 8.08 g

Fat: 5.97 g

Carbohydrates: 61.85 g

Chargrilled Beef with a Red Wine Jus, Onion Rings, Garlic Kale& Herb-Roasted Potatoes

Preparation time:

Cooking time:

Servings: 2

Ingredients

100 grams potatoes (peeled and cut into 2cm dice)

1 tbsp extra virgin olive oil

5g parsley, finely chopped

50g red onion, sliced into rings

50g Kale, sliced

1 garlic clove, finely chopped

120–150g x 3.5cm-thick beef fillet steak or 2cm-thick sirloin steak

40ml red wine

150ml beef stock

1 tsp tomato purée

1 tsp corn flour, dissolved in 1 tbsp water

Directions:

Heat your oven to 220°C/gas 7.

Place the potatoes in a saucepan with boiling water.

Bring back to the boil now cook for 4–5 minutes.

Drain.

Now place in a roasting tin with 1 teaspoon of the oil. Roast it in the hot oven for about 35 to 45 mins.

Turn the potatoes every 10 minutes.

When it is cooked, remove from the oven. Then sprinkle with the chopped parsley and mix well.

Fry the onion in 1 teaspoon oil and heat for 5 minutes. Fry till they get soft and nicely caramelized. Keep warm. Now steam the Kale for 2–3 minutes then drain.

Fry the garlic gently oil (1/2 tablespoon oil). Fry for one minute. It should get soft, but it should not be coloured. Add the Kale and fry for 2 minutes more, until it gets tender. Keep warm.

Heat a frying pan over high heat. Heat until smoking.

Coat the meat in ½ teaspoon of the oil, fry in the hot pan over a medium to high temperature, i.e. heat according to how you like your meat cooked.

If you like to cook the meat on a medium level, it would be better to sear the meat. Now transfer the pan to an oven set at 220°C/gas 7. Finish the cooking that way for a specific time.

Remove the meat from the pan. Set aside to rest. Now add the wine to the hot pan to bring up if any meat residue is left. Bubble to reduce the wine by its half. It becomes syrupy with a thick flavour in this way.

Add stock and tomato purée to the steak pan to boil it. Then keep adding the corn flour paste to thicken the sauce, adding it a little at a time until you have your desired thickness.

Stir in any of the juices from your steak.

Serve it with the roasted potatoes, Kale, onion rings and the red wine sauce.

Nutrition:

Calories: 240 kcal

Protein: 14.18 g

Fat: 14.42 g

Carbohydrates: 13.77 g

Buckwheat Pasta Salad

Preparation time: 30 minutes

Cooking time: 0 minutes

Servings 1

Ingredients

50g buckwheat pasta

large handful of rocket

a small handful of basil leaves

8 cherry tomatoes, halved

1/2 avocado, diced

10 olives

1 tbsp extra virgin olive oil

20g pine nuts

Directions:

Combine all the ingredients. Don't include the pine nuts. Arrange on a plate. Scatter the pine nuts over the top.

Nutrition:

Calories: 440 kcal

Protein: 6.82 g

Fat: 39.33 g

Carbohydrates: 22.48 g

Greek Salad Skewers

Preparation time: 45 minutes

Cooking time: 10 minutes

Servings: 2

Ingredients:

2 wooden skewers, soaked in water for 30 minutes before use

8 large black olives

8 cherry tomatoes

1 yellow pepper, cut into eight squares

½ red onion, chopped in half and separated into eight pieces

100g (about 10cm) cucumber, cut into four slices and halved

100g feta, cut into 8 cubes

For the dressing

1 tbsp extra virgin olive oil

Juice of ½ lemon

1 tsp balsamic vinegar

½ clove garlic, peeled and crushed

Few leaves of basil, finely chopped (or ½ tsp dried mixed herbs to replace basil and oregano)

Few leaves oregano (finely chopped)

generous seasoning of salt and ground black pepper

Directions:

First of all thread each skewer with the salad ingredients in the following order: - Olive, Tomato, Yellow pepper, Red onion, Cucumber, Feta, Tomato, Olive, Yellow pepper, Red onion, Cucumber, and Feta.

Now place all the dressing ingredients in a small bowl. Mix together and pour over the skewers.

Nutrition:

Calories: 287 kcal

Protein: 19.5 g

Fat: 17.45 g

Carbohydrates: 14.84 g

Kale, Edamame and Tofu Curry

Preparation time: 1 hour

Cooking time: 45 minutes

Servings: 4

Ingredients:

1 tbsp rapeseed oil

1 large onion, chopped

4 cloves garlic, peeled and grated

4 .1 large thumb (7cm) fresh ginger, peeled and grated

1 red chilli, deseeded and thinly sliced

1/2 tsp ground turmeric

1/4 tsp cayenne pepper

1 tsp paprika

1/2 tsp ground cumin

1 tsp salt

250g dried red lentils

1 litre boiling water

50g frozen soyaedamame beans

200g firm tofu, chopped into cubes

2 tomatoes, roughly chopped

Juice of 1 lime

200g kale leaves, stalks removed and torn

Directions:

Put the oil in a heavy-bottomed pan. Cook over low to medium heat. Add the onion in it and cook for 5 minutes.

Then add the garlic, ginger and chilli. After adding them and cook for two minutes.

Add turmeric, cayenne, paprika, cumin and salt. Stir through before you add the red lentils. Stir again.

Pour in the boiling water. Boil for 10 minutes. Now reduce the heat and cook for a further 20-30 minutes until the curry has a thick '•porridge' consistency.

Add the soya beans, tofu and tomatoes, cook for 5 minutes more. Add the lime juice and kale leaves. Cook until the Kale is just tender.

Nutrition:

Calories: 407 kcal

Protein: 27.67 g

Fat: 9.98 g

Carbohydrates: 57.95 g

Sirt Food Miso-Marinated Cod with Stir-Fried Greens and Sesame

Preparation time: 1 hour 10 minutes

Cooking time: 40 minutes

Servings: 1

Ingredients

20g miso

1 tbsp mirin

1 tbsp extra virgin olive oil

200g skinless cod fillet

20g red onion, sliced

40g celery, sliced

one garlic clove, finely chopped

one bird's eye chilli, finely chopped

1 tsp finely chopped fresh ginger

60g green beans

50g Kale, roughly chopped

1 tsp sesame seeds

5g parsley, roughly chopped

1 tbsp tamari

30g buckwheat

1 tsp ground turmeric

Directions:

Mix the miso and mirin with one teaspoon of the oil.

Rub all over cod and leave to marinate. Marinate for 30 minutes. Now heat the oven to 220°C/gas 7. Bake the cod for 10 minutes. Next heat a frying pan or wok with the remaining oil.

Add the onion to it and stir-fry for a few minutes. Add celery, garlic, chilli, ginger, green beans and Kale, all of them. Toss and fry until the Kale is tender and is cooked well, add a little water to the pan to aid the cooking process.

Cook the buckwheat according to the instructions on the packet. Cook it with turmeric for three minutes. Now add the sesame seeds, parsley and tamari to the stir-fry. Serve it with the greens and fish.

Nutrition:

Calories: 355 kcal

Protein: 40.31 g

Fat: 10.87 g

Carbohydrates: 25.94 g

Chocolate Bark

Preparation time: 30 minutes

Cooking time: 3 hours

Servings: 2

Ingredients:

1 thin peel orange

¾ cup pistachio nuts, roasted, chilled and chopped into large pieces

¼ cup hazelnuts, toasted, chilled, peeled and chopped into large pieces

¼ cup pumpkin seeds, toasted and chilled

1 tablespoon chia seeds

1 tablespoon sesame seeds, toasted and cooled

1 teaspoon grated orange peel

1 cardamom pod, finely crushed and sieved

12 ounces (340 g) tempered, dairy-free dark chocolate (65% cocoa content)

2 teaspoons flaky sea salt

Candy or candy thermometer

Directions:

Preheat the oven to 100-150 ° F (66 ° C). Line a baking sheet with parchment paper.

Finely slice the orange crosswise and place it on the prepared baking sheet. Bake for 2 to 3 hours until dry but slightly sticky. Remove it from the oven and let it cool.

When they cool enough to handle them, cut the orange slices into fragments; set them aside.

In a large bowl, mix the nuts, seeds, and grated orange peel until completely combined. Place the mixture in a single layer on a baking sheet lined with kitchen parchment. Set it aside.

Melt the chocolate in a water bath until it reaches 88 to 90 ° F (32 to 33 ° C) and pours it over the nut mixture to cover it completely.

When the chocolate is semi-cold but still sticky, sprinkle the surface with sea salt and pieces of orange.

Place the mixture in a cold area of your kitchen or refrigerate until the crust cools completely, and cut it into bite-sized pieces.

Nutrition:

Protein: 20.7 g

Calories: 523 kcal

Fat: 40.76 g

Carbohydrates: 26.65 g

Salmon and Spinach Quiche

Preparation time: 55 minutes

Cooking time: 45 minutes

Servings: 2

Ingredients:

600 g frozen leaf spinach

1 clove of garlic

1 onion

150 g frozen salmon fillets

200 g smoked salmon

1 small Bunch of dill

1 untreated lemon

50 g butter

200 g sour cream

3 eggs

Salt, pepper, nutmeg

1 pack of puff pastry

Directions:

Let the spinach thaw and squeeze well.

Peel the garlic and onion and cut into fine cubes.

Cut the salmon fillet into cubes 1-1.5 cm thick.

Cut the smoked salmon into strips.

Wash the dill, pat dry and chop.

Wash the lemon with hot water, dry, rub the zest finely with a kitchen grater and squeeze the lemon.

Heat the butter in a pan. Sweat the garlic and onion cubes in it for approx. 2-3 minutes.

Add spinach and sweat briefly.

Add sour cream, lemon juice and zest, eggs and dill and mix well.

Season with salt, pepper and nutmeg.

Preheat the oven to 200 degrees top / bottom heat (180 degrees convection).

Grease a springform pan and roll out the puff pastry in it and pull up on edge. Prick the dough with a fork (so that it doesn't rise too much).

Pour in the spinach and egg mixture and smooth out.

Spread salmon cubes and smoked salmon strips on top.

The quiche in the oven (grid, middle inset) about 30-40 min. Yellow gold bake.

Nutrition:

Calories: 903 kcal

Protein: 65.28 g

Fat: 59.79 g

Carbohydrates: 30.79 g

Turmeric Chicken & Kale Salad with Honey Lime Dressing

Preparation time: 55 minutes

Cooking time: 20 minutes

Servings: 2

Ingredients

For chicken

1 teaspoon ghee or 1 tablespoon of coconut oil

½ medium brown onion, diced

250-300 g / 9 oz. Ground chicken or cubed chicken thighs

1 large clove of garlic, finely diced

1 teaspoon turmeric powder

1 teaspoon lime zest

½ lime juice

½ tsp salt + pepper

For salad

6 stems of broccoli or 2 cups of broccoli florets

2 tablespoons of pumpkin seeds

3 large kale leaves, stems removed and chopped

½Avocado, slice

A handful of fresh coriander leaves, chopped

A handful of fresh parsley leaves chopped

dressing

3 tbsp lime juice

1 diced or grated small piece of garlic

3 tablespoons extra virgin olive oil

1 tsp raw honey

1/2 teaspoon whole grain

1/2 teaspoon sea salt

Pepper

Directions:

In a small frying pan, heat the ghee or coconut oil over medium to high heat. Add the onion and sauté for 4-5 minutes on medium heat, until golden. Attach the slimy chicken and garlic and swirl over medium-high heat for 2-3 minutes, breaking it apart.

Attach the turmeric, lime zest, lime juice, salt and pepper and cook for a further 3-4 minutes, stirring frequently. Set aside the cooked slush.

Bring a small saucepan of water to boil while the chicken cooks. Stir in the broccolini and cook 2 minutes. Rinse under cold water, and cut into three to four pieces each.

Throw the pumpkin seeds from the chicken into the frying pan and toast for 2 minutes over medium heat, stirring frequently to prevent burning. Season to a bit of salt. Deposit aside. Raw pumpkin seeds should also be used well.

In a salad bowl, place the chopped kale, and pour over the dressing. Toss the kale with the sauce, and rub it with your palms. This will soften the kale, kind of like what citrus juice does to carpaccio fish or beef–it' cooks' it a little bit.

The cooked rice, broccolini, fresh herbs, pumpkin seeds and slices of avocado are eventually tossed.

Nutrition:

Calories: 1290 kcal

Protein: 131.39 g

Fat: 66.95 g

Carbohydrates: 40.87 g

Buckwheat Noodles with Chicken Kale & Miso Dressing

Preparation time: 55 minutes

Cooking time: 20 minutes

Servings: 2

Ingredients:

For Noodles

2-3 handfuls of kale leaves (removed from the stem and roughly cut)

Buckwheat noodles 150 g / 5 oz (100% buckwheat, no wheat)

3-4 shiitake mushrooms, cut into slices

1 teaspoon of coconut oil or ghee

1 brown onion, finely diced

1 medium free-range chicken breast, sliced or cubed

1 long red chili, thinly chopped

2 large garlic cloves, finely diced

2-3 tablespoons of Tamari sauce (gluten-free soy sauce)

For miso dressing

1½ tbsp fresh organic miso

1 tbsp Tamari sauce

1 tablespoon of extra virgin olive oil

1 tablespoon lemon or lime juice

1 teaspoon sesame oil

Directions:

Bring a medium saucepan of boiling water. Attach the kale and cook until slightly wilted, for 1 minute. Remove and set aside, then bring the water back to the boil. Add the soba noodles and cook (usually about 5 minutes) according to packaging instructions. Set aside and rinse under cold water.

Meanwhile, in a little ghee or coconut oil (about a teaspoon), pan fry the shiitake mushrooms for 2-3 minutes, until lightly browned on either side. Sprinkle with salt from the sea, and set aside.

Heat more coconut oil or ghee in the same frying pan over medium to high heat. Stir in onion and chilli for 2-3 minutes, then add pieces of chicken. Cook over medium heat for 5 minutes, stirring a few times, then add the garlic, tamari sauce and some splash of water. Cook for another 2-3 minutes, always stirring until chicken is cooked through.

Eventually, add the kale and soba noodles and warm up by stirring through the food.

Right at the end of the cooking, mix the miso dressing and drizzle over the noodles, so you'll keep all those beneficial probiotics alive and active.

Nutrition:

Calories: 256 kcal

Protein: 10.82 g

Fat: 8.95 g

Carbohydrates: 37.03 g

Asian King Prawn Stir-Fry with Buckwheat Noodles

Preparation time: 55 minutes

Cooking time: 20 minutes

Servings: 2

Ingredients

150g raw royal shrimps in shelled skins

2 teaspoons of tamari (you can use soy sauce if you do not avoid gluten)

2 teaspoons extra virgin olive oil

75g soba (buckwheat noodles)

1 clove of garlic, finely chopped

1 aerial view of finely chopped chili

1 teaspoon of finely chopped fresh ginger

20g red onion, cut into slices

40g celery, trimmed and cut into slices

75g chopped green beans

50g kale, coarsely chopped

100 ml of chicken stock

5g lovage or celery leaves

Directions:

Heat a frying pan over high heat, then cook the prawns for 2–3 minutes in 1 teaspoon tamari and 1 teaspoon oil. Put the prawns on a plate. Wipe the pan out with paper from the oven, as you will be using it again.

Cook the noodles 5–8 minutes in boiling water, or as indicated on the packet. Drain and put away.

Meanwhile, over medium-high heat, fry the garlic, chili, and ginger, red onion, celery, beans and kale in the remaining oil for 2–3 minutes. Remove the stock and bring to the boil, then cook for one or two minutes until the vegetables are cooked but crunchy.

Add the prawns, noodles, and leaves of lovage/celery to the pan, bring back to the boil, then remove the heat and serve.

Nutrition:

Calories: 251 kcal

Protein: 22.97 g

Fat: 3.71 g

Carbohydrates: 34.14 g

Choc Chip Granola

Preparation time: 55 minutes

Cooking time: 20 minutes

Servings: 2

Ingredients:

200g large oat flakes

Roughly 50 g pecan nuts

chopped

3 tablespoons of light olive oil

20g butter

1 tablespoon of dark brown sugar

2 tbsp rice syrup

60 g of good quality (70%)

dark chocolate shavings

Directions:

Oven preheats to 160 ° C (140 ° C fan / Gas 3). Line a large baking tray with a sheet of silicone or parchment for baking.

In a large bowl, combine the oats and pecans. Heat the olive oil, butter, brown sugar, and rice malt syrup gently in a small non-stick pan until the butter has melted, and the sugar and syrup dissolve. Do not let boil. Pour the syrup over the oats and stir thoroughly until fully covered with the oats.

Spread the granola over the baking tray and spread right into the corners. Leave the mixture clumps with spacing, instead of even spreading. Bake for 20 minutes in the oven until golden brown is just tinged at the edges. Remove from the oven, and leave completely to cool on the tray.

When cold, split with your fingers any larger lumps on the tray and then mix them in the chocolate chips. Put the granola in an airtight tub or jar, or pour it. The granola is to last for at least 2 weeks.

Nutrition:

Calories: 914 kcal

Protein: 40.19 g

Fat: 63.05 g

Carbohydrates: 88.74 g

Fragrant Asian Hotpot

Preparation time: 30 minutes

Cooking time: 10 minutes

Servings: 2

Ingredients:

1 teaspoon tomato puree

1-star anise, crushed (or 1/4 teaspoon anise)

A small handful (10 g) of parsley, finely chopped stalks

A small handful of coriander (10 g), finely chopped stalks

Juice from 1/2 lime

500 ml chicken broth, fresh or made from 1 cube

1/2 carrot, peeled and cut into matches

50 g broccoli, cut into small roses

50 g bean sprouts

100 g raw tiger prawns

100 g hard tofu, chopped

50 g rice noodles, cooked according to the instructions on the packaging

50g of boiled water chestnuts, drained

20g chopped ginger sushi

1 tablespoon of good quality miso paste

Directions:

Place in a large saucepan the tomato purée, star anise, parsley stalks, coriander stalks, lime juice and chicken stock and bring 10 minutes to a simmer.

Stir in the cabbage, broccoli, prawns, tofu, noodles and water chestnuts and cook gently until the prawns are finished. Remove from heat and whisk in the ginger sushi and the paste miso.

Serve sprinkled with the leaves of the parsley and coriander.

Nutrition:

Calories: 253 kcal

Protein: 19.39 g

Fat: 7.35 g

Carbohydrates: 29.99 g

Sesame Chicken Salad

Preparation time: 30 minutes

Cooking time: 12 minutes

Servings: 2

Ingredients

1 tablespoon of sesame seeds

1 cucumber, peeled, deseeded and sliced

100g baby kale, roughly chopped

60g pak choi, finely shredded

½ red onion, finely sliced

20g parsley, chopped

150g cooked chicken, shredded

For the dressing:

1 tablespoon of extra virgin olive oil

1 teaspoon of sesame oil

1 lime

1 teaspoon of clear honey

2 teaspoons of soy sauce

Directions:

In a dry frying pan, put the sesame seeds and toast for 2 minutes to become lightly browned and fragrant. Put in a plate and set aside.

Put the olive oil, honey, soy sauce, sesame oil, and lime juice, in a small bowl and mix to make the dressing.

Put in a large bowl, the kale, cucumber, pak choi, parsley, and red onion and gently mix. Pour the dressing into the mixture and continue mixing.

Share the salad in two plates topping them with the shredded chicken. Sprinkle the sesame seeds and serve.

Nutrition:

Calories: 478 kcal

Protein: 19.53 g

Fat: 39.8 g

Carbohydrates: 12.52 g

Aromatic Chicken Breast, Kale, Red Onion, and Salsa

Preparation time: 55 minutes

Cooking time: 30 minutes

Servings: 2

Ingredients

120g skinless, boneless chicken breast

2 teaspoons ground turmeric

¼ lemon

1 tablespoon extra-virgin olive oil

50g kale, chopped

20g red onion, sliced

1 teaspoon fresh ginger, chopped

50g buckwheat

Directions:

To prepare the salsa, remove the tomato eye and finely chop. Add the chilli, parsley, capers, lemon juice and mix.

Preheat the oven to 220°C. Pour 1 teaspoon of the turmeric, the lemon juice and a little oil on the chicken breast and marinate. Allow to stay for 5–10 minutes.

Place an ovenproof frying pan on the heat and cook the marinated chicken for a minute on each side to achieve a pale golden colour. Then transfer the pan containing the chicken to the oven and allow to stay for 8–10 minutes or until it is done. Remove from the oven and cover with foil, set aside for 5 minutes before serving.

Put the kale in a steamer and cook for 5 minutes. Pour a little oil in a frying pan and fry the red onions and the ginger to become soft but not coloured. Add the cooked kale and continue to fry for another minute.

Cook the buckwheat following the packet's instructions using the remaining turmeric. Serve alongside the chicken, salsa, and vegetables.

Nutrition:

Calories: 149 kcal

Protein: 15.85 g

Fat: 5.09 g

Carbohydrates: 10.53 g

Kale and Red Onion Dhal with Buckwheat

Preparation time 5 minutes

Cooking time 25 minutes

Servings: 2

Ingredients

½ tablespoon olive oil

½ small red onion, sliced

1 ½ garlic cloves, crushed

1cm ginger, grated

½ birds eye chilli, deseeded and finely chopped

1 teaspoon turmeric

1 teaspoon garam masala

80g red lentils

200ml coconut milk

100ml water

50g kale or spinach

80g buckwheat or brown rice

Directions:

Heat up the olive oil, add the sliced onion and cook on a low heat for 5 minutes until softened with the lid on. Then, add the ginger, garlic, and chilli and continue cooking for extra 1 minute.

Add to it, the garam masala, turmeric, and a splash of water. Cook for 1 more minute before adding the coconut milk, red lentils, and 200ml water.

Thoroughly mix all together and cook over a gentle heat for 20 minutes with the lid closed. When the dhal starts sticking, add a little more water and stir occasionally.

Add the kale, after 20 minutes and thoroughly stir and still cover the lid to cook for additional 5 minutes or 1-2 minutes when you substitute with spinach.

Put the buckwheat in a saucepan and pour boiling water like 15 minutes before the curry gets ready. Allow the water to boil and cook for 10-12 minutes. Drain the buckwheat and serve with the dhal.

Nutrition:

Calories: 355 kcal

Protein: 14.39 g

Fat: 5.7 g

Carbohydrates: 63.41 g

Chargrilled Beef, A Red Wine Jus, Onion Rings, Garlic Kale, and Herb Roasted Potatoes

Preparation time: 1 hour 30 minutes

Cooking time: 1 hour 10 minutes

Servings: 2

Ingredients

100g potatoes, peeled and dice

1 tablespoon extra-virgin olive oil

5g parsley, finely chopped

50g red onion, sliced into rings

50g kale, sliced

1 garlic clove, finely chopped

120–150g x 3.5cm-thick beef fillet steak

40ml red wine 150ml beef stock

1 teaspoon tomato purée

1 teaspoon corn flour

1 tablespoon water

Directions:

Preheat the oven to 220°C and put the potatoes in a boiling water and cook for 4–5 minutes, drain. Pour 1 teaspoon oil in a roasting tin and roast the potatoes for 35–45 minutes turning the potatoes on every sides every 10 minutes to ensure they cook evenly.

Remove from the oven when fully cooked, sprinkle with chopped parsley and mix thoroughly.

Pour 1 teaspoon of the oil on a saucepan and fry the onion for 5-7 minutes to become soft and neatly caramelized. Keep it warm.

Place the kale in a saucepan, steam for 2–3 minutes and drain. In ½ teaspoon of oil, fry the garlic for 1 minute to become soft though not coloured. Add the kale and continue to fry for extra 1–2 minutes to become tender. Maintain the warmth.

Over a high heat, place an ovenproof frying pan until it becomes smoking. Then use the ½ a teaspoon of the oil to coat the meat and fry over a medium–high heat. Remove the meat and set aside to rest.

Pour the wine to the hot pan and bubble to reduce the wine quantity by half to form syrupy and to have a concentrated flavor. Add the tomato purée and stock to the steak pan and boil. Add the corn flour paste little at a time to act as a thickener to until the desired consistency is achieved. Add any juices from the rested steak and serve with the kale, onion rings, roasted potatoes, and red wine sauce.

Nutrition:

Calories: 244 kcal

Protein: 14.26 g

Fat: 14.46 g

Carbohydrates: 14.69 g

Braised Leek With Pine Nuts:

Preparation time: 45 minutes

Cooking time: 15 minutes

Servings: 2

Ingredients:

20 g Ghee

2 teaspoon Olive oil

2 pieces Leek

150 ml Vegetable broth

fresh parsley

1 tablespoon fresh oregano

1 tablespoon Pine nuts (roasted)

Directions:

Cut the leek into thin rings and finely chop the herbs. Roast the pine nuts in a dry pan over medium heat.

Melt the ghee together with the olive oil in a large pan.

Cook the leek until golden brown for 5 minutes, stirring constantly.

Add the vegetable broth and cook for another 10 minutes until the leek is tender.

Stir in the herbs and sprinkle the pine nuts on the dish just before serving.

Nutrition:

Calories: 95 kcal

Protein: 1.35 g

Fat: 4.84 g

Carbohydrates: 12.61 g

Sweet and Sour Pan with Cashew Nuts:

Preparation time: 30 minutes

Cooking time: 0 minutes

Servings: 2

Ingredients:

2 tablespoon Coconut oil

2 pieces Red onion

2 pieces yellow bell pepper

250 g White cabbage

150 g Pak choi

50 g Mung bean sprouts

4 pieces Pineapple slices

50 g Cashew nuts

For the sweet and sour sauce:

60 ml Apple cider vinegar

4 tablespoon Coconut blossom sugar

11/2 tablespoon Tomato paste

1 teaspoon Coconut-Aminos

2 teaspoon Arrowroot powder

75 ml Water

Directions:

Roughly cut the vegetables.

Mix the arrow root with five tablespoons of cold water into a paste.

Then put all the other ingredients for the sauce in a saucepan and add the arrowroot paste for binding.

Melt the coconut oil in a pan and fry the onion.

Add the bell pepper, cabbage, pak choi and bean sprouts and stir-fry until the vegetables become a little softer.

Add the pineapple and cashew nuts and stir a few more times.

Pour a little sauce over the wok dish and serve.

Nutrition:

Calories: 573 kcal

Protein: 15.25 g

Fat: 27.81 g

Carbohydrates: 77.91 g

Casserole with Spinach and Eggplant

Preparation time: 1 hour

Cooking time: 40 minutes

Servings: 2

Ingredients:

1 piece Eggplant

2 pieces Onion

Olive oil 3 tablespoon

Spinach (fresh) 450 g

Tomatoes 4 pieces

Egg 2 pieces

60 ml Almond milk

2 teaspoons Lemon juice

4 tablespoon Almond flour

Directions:

Preheat the oven to 200 ° C.

Cut the eggplants, onions and tomatoes into slices and sprinkle salt on the eggplant slices.

Brush the eggplants and onions with olive oil and fry them in a grill pan.

Shrink the spinach in a large saucepan over moderate heat and drain in a sieve.

Put the vegetables in layers in a greased baking dish: first the eggplant, then the spinach and then the onion and the tomato. Repeat this again.

Whisk eggs with almond milk, lemon juice, salt and pepper and pour over the vegetables.

Sprinkle almond flour over the dish and bake in the oven for about 30 to 40 minutes.

Nutrition:

Calories: 446 kcal

Protein: 13.95 g

Fat: 31.82 g

Carbohydrates: 30.5 g

Vegetarian Paleo Ratatouille:

Preparation time: 1 hour 10 minutes

Cooking time: 55 minutes

Servings: 2

Ingredients:

200 g Tomato cubes (can)

1/2 pieces Onion

2 cloves Garlic

1/4 teaspoon dried oregano

1 / 4 TL Chili flakes

2 tablespoon Olive oil

1 piece Eggplant

1 piece Zucchini

1 piece hot peppers

1 teaspoon dried thyme

Directions:

Preheat the oven to 180 ° C and lightly grease a round or oval shape.

Finely chop the onion and garlic.

Mix the tomato cubes with garlic, onion, oregano and chilli flakes, season with salt and pepper and put on the bottom of the baking dish.

Use a mandolin, a cheese slicer or a sharp knife to cut the eggplant, zucchini and hot pepper into very thin slices.

Put the vegetables in a bowl (make circles, start at the edge and work inside).

Drizzle the remaining olive oil on the vegetables and sprinkle with thyme, salt and pepper.

Cover the baking dish with a piece of parchment paper and bake in the oven for 45 to 55 minutes.

Enjoy it!

Nutrition:

Calories: 273 kcal

Protein: 5.66 g

Fat: 14.49 g

Carbohydrates: 35.81 g

Courgette and Broccoli Soup:

Preparation time: 20 minutes

Cooking time: 5 minutes

Servings: 2

Ingredients:

2 tablespoon Coconut oil

1 piece Red onion

2 cloves Garlic

300 g Broccoli

1 piece Zucchini

750 ml Vegetable broth

Directions:

Finely chop the onion and garlic, cut the broccoli into florets and the zucchini into slices.

Melt the coconut oil in a soup pot and fry the onion with the garlic.

Cook the zucchini for a few minutes.

Add broccoli and vegetable broth and simmer for about 5 minutes.

Puree the soup with a hand blender and season with salt and pepper.

Nutrition:

Calories: 178 kcal

Protein: 5.7 g

Fat: 14.43 g

Carbohydrates: 10.57 g

Frittata with Spring Onions and Asparagus:

Preparation time:

Cooking time:

Servings: 2

Ingredients:

5 pieces Egg

80 ml Almond milk

2 tablespoon Coconut oil

1 clove Garlic

100 g Asparagus tips

4 pieces Spring onions

1 teaspoon Tarragon

1 pinch Chilli flakes

Directions:

Preheat the oven to 220 ° C.

Squeeze the garlic and finely chop the spring onions.

Whisk the eggs with the almond milk and season with salt and pepper.

Melt 1 tablespoon of coconut oil in a medium-sized cast iron pan and briefly fry the onion and garlic with the asparagus.

Remove the vegetables from the pan and melt the remaining coconut oil in the pan.

Pour in the egg mixture and half of the entire vegetable.

Place the pan in the oven for 15 minutes until the egg has solidified.

Then take the pan out of the oven and pour the rest of the egg with the vegetables into the pan.

Place the pan in the oven again for 15 minutes until the egg is nice and loose.

Sprinkle the tarragon and chilli flakes on the dish before serving.

Nutrition:

Calories: 464 kcal

Protein: 24.23 g

Fat: 37.84 g

Carbohydrates: 7.33 g

Cucumber Salad with Lime and Coriander

Preparation time:

Cooking time:

Servings: 2

Ingredients:

1 piece Red onion

2 pieces Cucumber

2 pieces Lime (juice)

2 tablespoon fresh coriander

Directions:

Cut the onion into rings and thinly slice the cucumber. Chop the coriander finely.

Place the onion rings in a bowl and season with about half a tablespoon of salt.

Rub it in well and then fill the bowl with water.

Pour off the water and then rinse the onion rings thoroughly (in a sieve).

Put the cucumber slices together with onion, lime juice, coriander and olive oil in a salad bowl and stir everything well.

Season with a little salt.

You can keep this dish in the refrigerator in a covered bowl for a few days.

Nutrition:

Calories: 57 kcal

Protein: 2 g

Fat: 0.41 g

Carbohydrates: 13.22 g

Mexican Bell Pepper Filled With Egg:

Preparation time: 55 minutes

Cooking time: 20 minutes

Servings: 2

Ingredients:

1 tablespoon Coconut oil

4 pieces Egg

1 piece Tomato

1 pinch Chilli flakes

1/4 teaspoon Ground cumin

1/4 teaspoon Paprika powder

1/2 pieces Avocado

1 piece green peppers

2 tablespoon fresh coriander

Directions:

Cut the tomatoes and avocado into cubes and finely chop the fresh coriander.

Melt the coconut oil in a pan over medium heat, beat the eggs in the pan and add the tomato cubes.

Keep stirring until the eggs solidify and season with chilli, caraway, paprika, pepper, and salt.

Finally add the avocado.

Place the egg mixture in the pepper halves and garnish with fresh coriander.

Nutrition:

Calories: 497 kcal

Protein: 20.91 g

Fat: 41.27 g

Carbohydrates: 14.41 g

Honey Mustard Dressing

Preparation time: 10 minutes

Cooking time: 0 minutes

Servings: 2

Ingredients:

4 tablespoon Olive oil

11/2 teaspoon Honey

11/2 teaspoon Mustard

1 teaspoon Lemon juice

1 pinch Salt

Directions:

Mix olive oil, honey, mustard and lemon juice into an even dressing with a whisk.

Season with salt.

Nutrition:

Calories: 306 kcal

Protein: 0.58 g

Fat: 27.47 g

Carbohydrates: 16.96 g

Paleo Chocolate Wraps with Fruits

Preparation time: 25 minutes

Cooking time: 0 minutes

Servings: 2

Ingredients:

4 pieces Egg

100 ml Almond milk

2 tablespoons Arrowroot powder

4 tablespoons Chestnut flour

1 tablespoon Olive oil (mild)

2 tablespoons Maple syrup

2 tablespoons Cocoa powder

1 tablespoon Coconut oil

1 piece Banana

2 pieces Kiwi (green)

2 pieces Mandarins

Directions:

Mix all ingredients (except fruit and coconut oil) into an even dough.

Melt some coconut oil in a small pan and pour a quarter of the batter into it.

Bake it like a pancake baked on both sides.

Place the fruit in a wrap and serve it lukewarm.

A wonderfully sweet start to the day!

Nutrition:

Calories: 555 kcal

Protein: 20.09 g

Fat: 34.24 g

Carbohydrates: 45.62 g

Vegetarian Curry from the Crock Pot:

Preparation time: 6 hours 10 minutes

Cooking time: 6 hours

Servings: 2

Ingredients:

4 pieces Carrot

2 pieces Sweet potato

1 piece Onion

3 cloves Garlic

2 tablespoon Curry powder

1 teaspoon Ground caraway (ground)

1/4 teaspoon Chili powder

1/4 TL Celtic sea salt

1 pinch Cinnamon

100 ml Vegetable broth

400 g Tomato cubes (can)

250 g Sweet peas

2 tablespoon Tapioca flour

Directions:

Roughly chop vegetables and potatoes and press garlic. Halve the sugar snap peas.

Put the carrots, sweet potatoes and onions in the slow cooker.

Mix tapioca flour with curry powder, cumin, chili powder, salt and cinnamon and sprinkle this mixture on the vegetables.

Pour the vegetable broth over it.

Close the lid of the slow cooker and let it simmer for 6 hours on a low setting.

Stir in the tomatoes and sugar snap peas for the last hour.

Cauliflower rice is a great addition to this dish.

Nutrition:

Calories: 397 kcal

Protein: 9.35 g

Fat: 6.07 g

Carbohydrates: 81.55 g

Fried Cauliflower Rice:

Preparation time: 55 minutes

Cooking time: 10 minutes

Servings: 2

Ingredients:

1 piece Cauliflower

2 tablespoon Coconut oil

1 piece Red onion

4 cloves Garlic

60 ml Vegetable broth

1.5 cm fresh ginger

1 teaspoon Chili flakes

1/2 pieces Carrot

1/2 pieces Red bell pepper

1/2 pieces Lemon (the juice)

2 tablespoon Pumpkin seeds

2 tablespoon fresh coriander

Directions:

Cut the cauliflower into small rice grains in a food processor.

Finely chop the onion, garlic and ginger, cut the carrot into thin strips, dice the bell pepper and finely chop the herbs.

Melt 1 tablespoon of coconut oil in a pan and add half of the onion and garlic to the pan and fry briefly until translucent.

Add cauliflower rice and season with salt.

Pour in the broth and stir everything until it evaporates and the cauliflower rice is tender.

Take the rice out of the pan and set it aside.

Melt the rest of the coconut oil in the pan and add the remaining onions, garlic, ginger, carrots and peppers.

Fry for a few minutes until the vegetables are tender. Season them with a little salt.

Add the cauliflower rice again, heat the whole dish and add the lemon juice.

Garnish with pumpkin seeds and coriander before serving.

Nutrition:

Calories: 230 kcal

Protein: 5.13 g

Fat: 17.81 g

Carbohydrates: 17.25 g

Mediterranean Paleo Pizza:

Preparation time: 55 minutes

Cooking time: 25 minutes

Servings: 2

Ingredients:

For the pizza crusts:

120 g Tapioca flour

1 teaspoon Celtic sea salt

2 tablespoon Italian spice mix

45 g Coconut flour

120 ml Olive oil (mild)

Water (warm) 120 ml

Egg (beaten) 1 piece

For covering:

2 tablespoon Tomato paste (can)

1/2 pieces Zucchini

1/2 pieces Eggplant

2 pieces Tomato

2 tablespoon Olive oil (mild)

1 tablespoon Balsamic vinegar

Directions:

Preheat the oven to 190 ° C and line a baking sheet with parchment paper.

Cut the vegetables into thin slices.

Mix the tapioca flour with salt, Italian herbs and coconut flour in a large bowl.

Pour in olive oil and warm water and stir well.

Then add the egg and stir until you get an even dough.

If the dough is too thin, add 1 tablespoon of coconut flour at a time until it is the desired thickness. Always wait a few minutes before adding more coconut flour, as it will take some time to absorb the moisture. The intent is to get a soft, sticky dough.

Divide the dough into two parts and spread them in flat circles on the baking sheet (or make 1 large sheet of pizza as shown in the picture).

Bake in the oven for about 10 minutes.

Brush the pizza with tomato paste and spread the aubergines, zucchini and tomato overlapping on the pizza.

Drizzle the pizza with olive oil and bake in the oven for another 10-15 minutes.

Drizzle balsamic vinegar over the pizza before serving.

Nutrition:

Calories: 574 kcal

Protein: 16.82 g

Fat: 25.92 g

Carbohydrates: 70.11 g

Fried Chicken and Broccolini:

Preparation time:

Cooking time:

Servings: 2

Ingredients:

2 tablespoon Coconut oil

400 g Chicken breast

Bacon cubes 150 g

Broccolini 250 g

Directions:

Cut the chicken into cubes.

Melt the coconut oil in a pan over medium heat and brown the chicken with the bacon cubes and cook through.

Season with chili flakes, salt and pepper.

Add broccolini and fry.

Stack on a plate and enjoy!

Nutrition:

Calories: 461 kcal

Protein: 41.7 g

Fat: 32.1 g

Carbohydrates: 4 g

Raw Vegan Walnuts Pie Crust & Raw Brownies

Preparation time: 5 Minutes

Cooking time: 40 Minutes

Servings 2

Ingredients

1 1/2 cups walnuts

1 cup pitted dates

1 1/2 tsp. ground vanilla bean

1/3 cup unsweetened cocoa powder

Topping for Raw Brownies:

1/3 cup walnut butter

Directions

Add walnuts to a food processor or blender. Mix until finely ground.

Add the vanilla, dates, and cocoa powder to the blender. Mix well and optionally add a couple drops of water at a time to make the mixture stick together.

This is a basic Raw Walnuts Pie Crust recipe.

If you need pie crust than spread it thinly in a 9 inch disc and add filling.

If you want to make Raw Brownies, than transfer the mixture into a small dish and top with walnut butter.

Nutrition:

Calories: 899 kcal

Protein: 13.83 g

Fat: 71.65 g

Carbohydrates: 71.67 g

Carrot, Buckwheat, Tomato & Arugula Salad in a Jar

Preparation time: 5 Minutes

Cooking Time: 30 Minutes

Servings 2

Ingredients

1/2 cup sunflower seeds

1/2 cup carrots

1/2 cup of shredded cabbage

1/2 cup of tomatoes

1 cup cooked buckwheat mixed with 1 tbsp. chia seeds

1 cup arugula

Dressing:

1 tbsp. olive oil

1 tbsp. fresh lemon juice and pinch of sea salt

Directions:

Put ingredients in this order: dressing, sunflower seeds, carrots, cabbage, tomatoes, buckwheat and arugula.

Nutrition:

Calories: 293 kcal

Protein: 8.46 g

Fat: 25.02 g

Carbohydrates: 13.62 g

Chickpeas, Onion, Tomato & Parsley Salad in a Jar

Preparation time: 5 Minutes

Cooking Time: 50 Minutes

Servings 2

Ingredients

1 cup cooked chickpeas

1/2 cup chopped tomatoes

1/2 of a small onion, chopped

1 tbsp. chia seeds

1 Tbsp. chopped parsley

Dressing:

1 tbsp. olive oil and 1 tbsp. of Chlorella.

1 tbsp. fresh lemon juice and pinch of sea salt

Directions:

Put ingredients in this order: dressing, tomatoes, chickpeas, onions and parsley.

Nutrition:

Calories: 210 kcal

Protein: 7.87 g

Fat: 9 g

Carbohydrates: 26.22 g

Kale & Feta Salad with Cranberry Dressing

Preparation time: 5 Minutes

Cooking Time: 30 Minutes

Servings 2

Ingredients

9oz kale, finely chopped

2oz walnuts, chopped

3oz feta cheese, crumbled

1 apple, peeled, cored and sliced

4 medjool dates, chopped

For the Dressing

3oz cranberries

½ red onion, chopped

3 tablespoons olive oil

3 tablespoons water

2 teaspoons honey

1 tablespoon red wine vinegar

Sea salt

Directions

Place the ingredients for the dressing into a food processor and process until smooth. If it seems too thick you can add a little extra water if necessary. Place all the ingredients for the salad into a bowl. Pour on the dressing and toss the salad until it is well coated in the mixture.

Nutrition:

Calories: 706 kcal

Protein: 15.62 g

Fat: 45.92 g

Carbohydrates: 70.28 g

Tuna, Egg & Caper Salad

Preparation time: 5 Minutes

Cooking Time: 20 Minutes

Servings 2

Ingredients

3½ozred chicory or yellow if not available

5oz tinned tuna flakes in brine, drained

3 ½ oz cucumber

1oz rocket arugula

6 pitted black olives

2 hard-boiled eggs, peeled and quartered

2 tomatoes, chopped

2 tablespoons fresh parsley, chopped

1 red onion, chopped

1 stalk of celery

1 tablespoon capers

2 tablespoons garlic vinaigrette see recipe

Directions

Place the tuna, cucumber, olives, tomatoes, onion, chicory, celery, parsley and rocket arugula into a bowl. Pour in the vinaigrette and toss the salad in the dressing. Serve onto plates and scatter the eggs and capers on top.

Nutrition:

Calories: 309 kcal

Protein: 26.72 g

Fat: 12.23 g

Carbohydrates: 25.76 g

Strawberry Buckwheat Pancakes

Preparation time: 5 Minutes

Cooking Time: 45 Minutes

Servings 4

Ingredients

3½oz strawberries, chopped

3½ oz buckwheat flour

1 egg

8fl oz milk

1 teaspoon olive oil

1 teaspoon olive oil for frying

Freshly squeezed juice of 1 orange

Directions

Pour the milk into a bowl and mix in the egg and a teaspoon of olive oil. Sift in the flour to the liquid mixture until smooth and creamy. Allow it to rest for 15 minutes. Heat a little oil in a pan and pour in a quarter of the mixture or to the size you prefer.

Sprinkle in a quarter of the strawberries into the batter. Cook for around 2 minutes on each side. Serve hot with a drizzle of orange juice. You could try experimenting with other berries such as blueberries and blackberries.

Nutrition:

Calories: 180 kcal

Protein: 7.46 g

Fat: 7.5 g

Carbohydrates: 22.58 g

Dal with Kale, Red Onions and Buckwheat

Preparation time: 5 Minutes

Cooking Time: 20 Minutes

Servings 2

Ingredients

1 teaspoon of extra virgin olive oil

1 teaspoon of mustard seeds

40g red onions, finely chopped

1 clove of garlic, very finely chopped

1 teaspoon very finely chopped ginger

1 Thai chili, very finely chopped

1 teaspoon curry mixture

2 teaspoons turmeric

300ml vegetable broth

40g red lentils

50g kale, chopped

50ml coconut milk

50g buckwheat

Directions

Heat oil in a pan at medium temperature and add mustard seeds. When they crack, add onion, garlic, ginger and chili. Heat until everything is soft.

Add the curry powder and 1 teaspoon of turmeric, mix well.

Add the vegetable stock, bring to the boil.

Add the lentils and cook them for 25 to 30 minutes until they are ready.

Then add the kale and coconut milk and simmer for 5 minutes. The Dal is ready.

While the lentils are cooking, prepare the buckwheat.

Serve buckwheat with the dal.

Nutrition:

Calories: 143 kcal

Protein: 7.67 g

Fat: 2.41 g

Carbohydrates: 24.83 g

Pancakes with Apples and Blackcurrants

Preparation time: 5 Minutes

Cooking Time: 50 Minutes

Servings 4

Ingredients

2 apples, cut into small chunks

2 cups of quick cooking oats

1 cup flour of your choice

1 tsp baking powder

2 tbsp. raw sugar, coconut sugar, or 2 tbsp. honey that is warm and easy to distribute

2 egg whites

1 ¼ cups of milk or soy/rice/coconut

2 tsp extra virgin olive oil

A dash of salt

For the berry topping:

1 cup blackcurrants, washed and stalks removed

3 tbsp. water may use less

2 tbsp. sugar see above for types

Directions

Place the ingredients for the topping in a small pot simmer, stirring frequently for about 10 minutes until it cooks down and the juices are released.

Take the dry ingredients and mix in a bowl. After, add the apples and the milk a bit at a time you may not use it all), until it is a batter. Stiffly whisk the egg whites and then gently mix them into the pancake batter. Set aside in the refrigerator.

Pour a one quarter of the oil onto a flat pan or flat griddle, and when hot, pour some of the batter into it in a pancake shape. When the pancakes start to have golden brown edges and form air bubbles, they may be ready to be gently flipped.

Test to be sure the bottom can life away from the pan before actually flipping. Repeat for the next three pancakes. Top each pancake with the berries.

Nutrition:

Calories: 470 kcal

Protein: 11.71 g

Fat: 16.83 g

Carbohydrates: 79 g

Miso Caramelized Tofu

Preparation time: 55 minutes

Cooking time: 15 minutes

Servings: 2

Ingredients

1 tbsp mirin

20g miso paste

1 * 150g firm tofu

40g celery, trimmed

35g red onion

120g courgette

1 bird's eye chili

1 garlic clove, finely chopped

1 tsp finely chopped fresh ginger

50g kale, chopped

2 tsp sesame seeds

35g buckwheat

1 tsp ground turmeric

2 tsp extra virgin olive oil

1 tsp tamari (or soy sauce)

Directions

Pre-heat your over to 200C or gas mark 6. Cover a tray with baking parchment.

Combine the mirin and miso together. Dice the tofu and coat it in the mirin-miso mixture in a resealable plastic bag. Set aside to marinate.

Chop the vegetables (except for the kale) at a diagonal angle to produce long slices. Using a steamer, cook for the kale for 5 minutes and set aside.

Disperse the tofu across the lined tray and garnish with sesame seeds. Roast for 20 minutes, or until caramelized.

Rinse the buckwheat using running water and a sieve. Add to a pan of boiling water alongside turmeric and cook the buckwheat according to the packet instructions.

Heat the oil in a skillet over high heat. Toss in the vegetables, herbs and spices then fry for 2-3 minutes. Reduce to a medium heat and fry for a further 5 minutes or until cooked but still crunchy.

Nutrition:

Calories: 101 kcal

Protein: 4.22 g

Fat: 4.7 g

Carbohydrates: 12.38 g

Sirtfood Cauliflower Couscous & Turkey Steak

Preparation time: 45 minutes

Cooking time: 10 minutes

Servings: 2

Ingredients:

150g cauliflower, roughly chopped

1 garlic clove, finely chopped

40g red onion, finely chopped

1 bird's eye chili, finely chopped

1 tsp finely chopped fresh ginger

2 tbsp extra virgin olive oil

2 tsp ground turmeric

30g sun dried tomatoes, finely chopped

10g parsley

150g turkey steak

1 tsp dried sage

Juice of ½ lemon

1 tbsp capers

Directions:

Disintegrate the cauliflower using a food processor. Blend in 1-2 pulses until the cauliflower has a breadcrumb-like consistency.

In a skillet, fry garlic, chili, ginger and red onion in 1 tsp olive oil for 2-3 minutes. Throw in the turmeric and cauliflower then cook for another 1-2 minutes. Remove from heat and add the tomatoes and roughly half the parsley.

Garnish the turkey steak with sage and dress with oil. In a skillet, over medium heat, fry the turkey steak for 5 minutes, turning occasionally. Once the steak is cooked add lemon juice, capers and a dash of water. Stir and serve with the couscous.

Nutrition:

Calories: 462 kcal

Protein: 16.81 g

Fat: 39.86 g

Carbohydrates: 9.94 g

Tuna Salad

Preparation time: 30 minutes

Cooking time: 0 minutes

Servings: 2

Ingredients:

100g red chicory

150g tuna flakes in brine, drained

100g cucumber

25g rocket

6 kalamata olives, pitted

2 hard-boiled eggs, peeled and quartered

2 tomatoes, chopped

2 tbsp fresh parsley, chopped

1 red onion, chopped

1 celery stalk

1 tbsp capers

2 tbsp garlic vinaigrette

Directions:

Combine all ingredients in a bowl and serve.

Nutrition:

Calories: 308 kcal

Protein: 27.13 g

Fat: 12.2 g

Carbohydrates: 24.6 g

Tofu & Shiitake Mushroom Soup

Preparation time: 30 minutes

Cooking time: 3 minutes

Servings: 4

Ingredients:

10g dried wakame

1L vegetable stock

200g shiitake mushrooms, sliced

120g miso paste

1* 400g firm tofu, diced

2 green onion, trimmed and diagonally chopped

1 bird's eye chili, finely chopped

Directions:

Soak the wakame in lukewarm water for 10-15 minutes before draining.

In a medium-sized saucepan add the vegetable stock and bring to the boil. Toss in the mushrooms and simmer for 2-3 minutes.

Mix miso paste with 3-4 tbsp of vegetable stock from the saucepan, until the miso is entirely dissolved. Pour the miso-stock back into the pan and add the tofu, wakame, green onions and chili, then serve immediately.

Nutrition:

Calories: 99 kcal

Protein: 4.75 g

Fat: 2.12 g

Carbohydrates: 17.41 g

Mushroom & Tofu Scramble

Preparation time: 30 minutes

Cooking time: 15 minutes

Servings: 1

Ingredients:

100g tofu, extra firm

1 tsp ground turmeric

1 tsp mild curry powder

20g kale, roughly chopped

1 tsp extra virgin olive oil

20g red onion, thinly sliced

50g mushrooms, thinly sliced

5g parsley, finely chopped

Directions:

Place 2 sheets of kitchen towel under and on-top of the tofu, then rest a considerable weight such as saucepan onto the tofu, to ensure it drains off the liquid.

Combine the curry powder, turmeric and 1-2 tsp of water to form a paste. Using a steamer cook kale for 3-4 minutes.

In a skillet, warm oil over a medium heat. Add the chili, mushrooms and onion, cooking for several minutes or until brown and tender.

Break the tofu in to small pieces and toss in the skillet. Coat with the spice paste and stir, ensuring everything becomes evenly coated. Cook for up to 5 minutes, or until the tofu has browned then add the kale and fry for 2 more minutes. Garnish with parsley before serving.

Nutrition:

Calories: 333 kcal

Protein: 20.49 g

Fat: 22.89 g

Carbohydrates: 18.83 g

Prawn & Chili Pak Choi

Preparation time: 30 minutes

Cooking time: 15 minutes

Servings: 1

Ingredients:

75g brown rice

1 pak choi

60ml chicken stock

1 tbsp extra virgin olive oil

1 garlic clove, finely chopped

50g red onion, finely chopped

½ bird's eye chili, finely chopped

1 tsp freshly grated ginger

125g shelled raw king prawns

1 tbsp soy sauce

1 tsp five-spice

1 tbsp freshly chopped flat-leaf parsley

A pinch of salt and pepper

Directions:

Bring a medium sized saucepan of water to the boil and cook the brown rice for 25-30 minutes, or until softened.

Tear the pak choi into pieces. Warm the chicken stock in a skillet over medium heat and toss in the pak choi, cooking until the pak choi has slightly wilted.

In another skillet, warm olive oil over high heat. Toss in the ginger, chili, red onions and garlic frying for 2-3 minutes.

Throw in the pawns, five-spice and soy sauce and cook for 6-8 minutes, or until the cooked throughout. Drain the brown rice and add to the skillet, stirring and cooking for 2-3 minutes. Add the pak choi, garnish with parsley and serve.

Nutrition:

Calories: 403 kcal

Protein: 16.15 g

Fat: 15.28 g

Carbohydrates: 50.87 g

Sirtfood Granola

Preparation time: 1 hour 10 minutes

Cooking time: 50 minutes

Servings: 12

Ingredients:

200g oats

250g buckwheat flakes

100g walnuts, chopped

100g almonds, chopped

100g dried strawberries

1 ½ tsp ground ginger

1 ½ tsp ground cinnamon

120mls olive oil

2 tbsp honey

Directions:

Preheat oven to 150C or gas mark 3. Line a tray with baking parchment.

Stir together walnuts, almonds, buckwheat flakes and oats with ginger and cinnamon. In a large pan, warm olive oil and honey, heating until the honey has dissolved.

Pour the honey-oil over the other ingredients, stirring to ensuring an even coating. Separate the granola evenly over the lined baking tray and roast for 50 minutes, or until golden.

Remove from the oven and leave to cool. Once cooled add the berries and store in an airtight container. Eat dry or with milk and yogurt. It stays fresh for up to 1 week.

Nutrition:

Calories: 178 kcal

Protein: 6.72 g

Fat: 10.93 g

Carbohydrates: 22.08 g

Tomato Frittata

Preparation time: 55 minutes

Cooking time: 20 minutes

Servings: 2

Ingredients:

50g cheddar cheese, grated

75g kalamata olives, pitted and halved

8 cherry tomatoes, halved

4 large eggs

1 tbsp fresh parsley, chopped

1 tbsp fresh basil, chopped

1 tbsp olive oil

Directions:

Whisk eggs together in a large mixing bowl. Toss in the parsley, basil, olives, tomatoes and cheese, stirring thoroughly.

In a small skillet, heat the olive oil over high heat. Pour in the frittata mixture and cook for 5-10 minutes, or set. Remove the skillet from the hob and place under the grill for 5 minutes, or until firm and set. Divide into portions and serve immediately.

Nutrition:

Calories: 269 kcal

Protein: 9.23 g

Fat: 23.76 g

Carbohydrates: 5.49 g

Horseradish Flaked Salmon Fillet & Kale

Preparation time: 55 minutes

Cooking time: 30 minutes

Servings: 2

Ingredients:

200g skinless, boneless salmon fillet

50g green beans

75g kale

1 tbsp extra virgin olive oil

½ garlic clove, crushed

50g red onion, chopped

1 tbsp fresh chives, chopped

1 tbsp freshly chopped flat-leaf parsley

1 tbsp low fat crème fraiche

1tbsp horseradish sauce

Juice of ¼ lemon

A pinch of salt and pepper

Directions:

Preheat the grill.

Sprinkle a salmon fillet with salt and pepper. Place under the grill for 10-15 minutes. Flake and set aside.

Using a steamer, cook the kale and green beans for 10 minutes.

In a skillet, warm the oil over a high heat. Add garlic and red onion and fry for 2-3 minutes. Toss in the kale and beans, and then cook for 1-2 minutes more.

Mix the chives, parsley, crème fraiche, horseradish, lemon juice and flaked salmon.

Serve the kale and beans topped with the dressed flaked salmon.

Nutrition:

Calories: 206 kcal

Protein: 26.7 g

Fat: 6.5 g

Carbohydrates: 11.12 g

Sirtfood Scrambled Eggs

Preparation time: 30 minutes

Cooking time: 10 minutes

Servings: 1

Ingredients:

1 tsp extra virgin olive oil

20g red onion, finely chopped

½ bird's eye chili, finely chopped

3 medium eggs

50ml milk

1 tsp ground turmeric

5g parsley, finely chopped

Directions:

In a skillet, heat the oil over a high heat. Toss in the red onion and chili, frying for 2-3 minutes.

In a large bowl, whisk together the milk, parsley, eggs and turmeric. Pour into the skillet and lower to medium heat. Cook for 3 to 5 minutes, scrambling the mixture as you do with a spoon or spatula. Serve immediately.

Nutrition:

Calories: 224 kcal

Protein: 17.2 g

Fat: 14.63 g

Carbohydrates: 4.79 g

Chicken Thighs with Creamy Tomato Spinach Sauce

Preparation time: 45 minutes

Cooking time: 10 minutes

Servings: 2

Ingredients:

One tablespoon olive oil

1.5 lb. chicken thighs, boneless skinless

1/2 teaspoon salt

1/4 teaspoon pepper

8 Oz tomato sauce

Two garlic cloves, minced

1/2 cup overwhelming cream

4 Oz new spinach

Four leaves fresh basil (or utilize 1/4 teaspoon dried basil)

Directions:

The most effective method to cook boneless skinless chicken thighs in a skillet: In a much skillet heat olive oil on medium warmth. Boneless chicken with salt and pepper. Add top side down to the hot skillet. Cook for 5 minutes on medium heat, until the high side, is pleasantly burned.

Flip over to the opposite side and heat for five additional minutes on medium heat. Expel the chicken from the skillet to a plate. Step by step instructions to make creamy tomato basil sauce: To the equivalent, presently void skillet, include tomato sauce, minced garlic, substantial cream. Bring to bubble and mix. Lessen warmth to low stew. Include new spinach and new basil. Mix until spinach withers and diminishes in volume. Taste the sauce and include progressively salt and pepper, if necessary. Include back cooked boneless skinless chicken thighs, increment warmth to medium.

Nutrition:

Calories: 1061 kcal

Protein: 66.42 g

Fat: 77.08 g

Carbohydrates: 29.51 g

Creamy Beef and Shells

Preparation time: 45 minutes

Cooking time: 20 minutes

Servings: 2

Ingredients:

8 ounces medium pasta shells

One tablespoon olive oil

1 pound ground meat

One little sweet onion (diced)

Five cloves garlic (minced)

One teaspoon Italian flavouring

One teaspoon dried parsley

1/2 teaspoon dried oregano

1/2 teaspoon smoked paprika

Two tablespoons generally useful flour

1 cup meat stock

1 (15oz can) marinara sauce

3/4 cup overwhelming cream

1/4 cup sharp cream

Legitimate salt and crisply ground dark pepper (to taste)

1/2 cups cheddar (newly ground)

Directions:

Cook pasta as per bundle directions in an enormous pot of bubbling salted water and channel well. W olive oil in a large skillet over medium-high warmth. Include ground meat and cook until caramelized, around 3-5 minutes, breaking it with a wooden spoon. Channel abundance fat and put in a safe spot. To a similar skillet, include diced onion, and cook for 2minutes, mixing now and again. Include garlic, and cook until fragrant, around one moment. Speed in flour until delicately caramelized, for around one moment. Step by step rush in hamburger stock and mix to join. Include marinara sauce and mix in Italian flavouring, dried parsley, oregano, and paprika. Heat to the boiling point, diminish warmth and stew, mixing once in a while until decreased and somewhat thickened around 6-8 minutes. Mix in cooked pasta, include back meat. Mix in overwhelming cream until warmed through, about 1-2 minutes. Taste and change for salt and pepper. Mix in sour cream. Mix in cheddar until liquefied, about 1-2 minutes. Serve promptly, embellish with parsley whenever wanted.

Nutrition:

Calories: 1196 kcal

Protein: 81.68 g

Fat: 61.32 g

Carbohydrates: 88.46 g

Shrimp Pasta

Preparation time: 45 minutes

Cooking time: 10 minutes

Servings: 2

Ingredients:

8 ounces linguine

1/4 cup mayonnaise

1/4 cup bean stew glue

Two cloves garlic, squashes

1/2 pound shrimp, stripped

One teaspoon salt

1/2 teaspoon cayenne pepper

One teaspoon garlic powder

One tablespoon vegetable oil

One lime, squeezed

1/4 cup green onion, slashed

1/4 cup cilantro, minced

Red bean stew chips, for embellish

Directions:

Cook pasta still somewhat firm as per box guidelines. In a little bowl, consolidate mayonnaise, stew glue and garlic. Race to join. Put in a safe spot. In a blending bowl, include shrimp, salt, cayenne and garlic powder. Mix to cover shrimp. Oil in a heavy skillet over medium warmth. Include shrimp and cook for around 2 minutes at that point flip and cook for an extra 2 minutes. Add pasta and sauce to the dish. Mood killer the warmth and combine until the pasta is covered. Include lime, green onions and cilantro, and topped with red bean stew pieces.

Nutrition:

Calories: 283 kcal

Protein: 25.75 g

Fat: 18.04 g

Carbohydrates: 6.07 g

Creamy Shrimp & Mozzarella Pasta

Preparation time: 45 minutes

Cooking time: 10 minutes

Servings: 2

Ingredients:

2 cups penne pasta, cooked still somewhat firm

Two tablespoons olive oil

Four cloves garlic, minced

1 pound shrimp, stripped and deveined

Two teaspoons salt, partitioned

1/2 cups substantial cream

1 cup destroyed mozzarella

1/2 cup sun-dried tomatoes

Two tablespoons cleaved basil

1/2 teaspoon red pepper pieces

Two teaspoons lemon juice

Cleaved basil, to decorate

Directions:

In a heavy skillet over medium-high warmth, saute garlic in olive oil until fragrant, around 2 minutes. Include shrimp and cook about 3 minutes on each side. Season with a large portion of the salt, expel from skillet and put in a safe spot. In a similar skillet, add overwhelming cream and heat to the point of boiling. Diminish to a stew and include mozzarella, sun-dried tomatoes, basil and red pepper chips. Stew for 5 minutes and lessen to low warmth. Return shrimp to the dish and include lemon squeeze and staying salt. Include cooked pasta and basil and serve.

Nutrition:

Calories: 664 kcal

Protein: 70.86 g

Fat: 20.94 g

Carbohydrates: 51.53 g

Beef Stroganoff French Bread Toast

Preparation time:

Cooking time:

Servings: 2

Ingredients:

4 tablespoons olive oil

1/2 cups mushrooms

2 teaspoons salt, separated

1/2 teaspoon dark pepper

2 tablespoons thyme

2 tablespoons spread

1/2 cup onions, diced

2 cloves garlic, minced

1 pound ground meat

3 tablespoons generally useful flour

2 teaspoons paprika

1/2 cups meat juices

1/2 cup sharp cream

1 teaspoon Dijon mustard

For the toasts:

1 portion French bread, inner parts dugout

2 cups mozzarella

3 tablespoons cleaved Italian parsley

Directions:

Preheat stove to 350 degrees, and line a sheet container with material paper. Make the stroganoff: In a large Dutch grill or skillet, heat olive oil over medium warmth. Saute mushrooms with one teaspoon salt and dark pepper. Include thyme. Cook mushrooms until brilliant, roughly 4 minutes. Expel from a dish and put in a safe spot. Include margarine, onions and garlic to the container and saute 2 minutes. Cook ground hamburger over medium warmth until dark-coloured, roughly 4 minutes. Add flour and paprika to cover uniformly. Include meat soup, sour cream and mustard. Blend entirely and include mushrooms back in. Round the emptied portion with stroganoff and top with mozzarella cheddar. Spot on the readied heating sheet, and prepare for 5 to 10 minutes until cheddar is brilliant and softened. Head with parsley, cut and serve right away.

Nutrition:

Calories: 1007 kcal

Protein: 88.04 g

Fat: 60 g

Carbohydrates: 32.06 g

Conclusion

Over the course of this book, you have not only learned the basic information required to start the Sirtfood diet, but you have also gained much more than that! By learning how to meal plan, prep, and storage, you will be able to easily master the Sirt food diet with little day-to-day effort required. You will be able to enjoy delicious meals at a moment's notice without having to struggle after a long day of work. By just preparing a little ahead of time, you can have a fridge and freezer fully stocked with delicious homemade meals perfectly suited to your taste.

The menu plan I provided you will help you get on your feet. Whether you choose to use the plan exactly how I designed, customize it, or create your own from scratch, you will find that by having a plan and guide to follow eating healthier, losing weight and boosting your health can be easier than ever.

There are over eighty recipes in this book, all of which can help you along every step of your journey to reach your goal. Whether your favorite recipe is Fudgy Buckwheat Brownies, Mulled Wine, Gluten-Free Buckwheat Pancakes, BBQ Tempeh Sandwiches, or Chicken with Balsamic Onions and Mushrooms, you are sure to find a number of dishes that you love.

Whether you start out following the Sirt diet to the letter or simply experimenting and enjoying the dishes in this book, you are sure to experience benefits and fall in love with food all over again. What are you waiting for? With just a little effort and time in the kitchen, you can get on your way to success.

Thank you for reading this book! I hope that you find the success you are looking for. If you enjoy the delicious recipes in this book, then be sure to look for my book Sirt Diet so that you can gain more valuable information and insight into the Sirt diet.

Made in the USA
Middletown, DE
14 May 2020